# Cutting-Edge in Arthroplasty:
# Before, While and after Surgery

# Cutting-Edge in Arthroplasty: Before, While and after Surgery

Editor

**Johannes Beckmann**

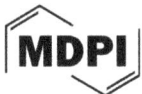

Basel • Beijing • Wuhan • Barcelona • Belgrade • Novi Sad • Cluj • Manchester

*Editor*
Johannes Beckmann
Department of Orthopedic
Surgery and Traumatology
Hospital Barmherzige Brüder Munich
München
Germany

*Editorial Office*
MDPI
St. Alban-Anlage 66
4052 Basel, Switzerland

This is a reprint of articles from the Special Issue published online in the open access journal *Journal of Personalized Medicine* (ISSN 2075-4426) (available at: www.mdpi.com/journal/jpm/special_issues/cutting_edge_arthroplasty).

For citation purposes, cite each article independently as indicated on the article page online and as indicated below:

Lastname, A.A.; Lastname, B.B. Article Title. *Journal Name* **Year**, *Volume Number*, Page Range.

**ISBN 978-3-7258-0660-7 (Hbk)**
**ISBN 978-3-7258-0659-1 (PDF)**
doi.org/10.3390/books978-3-7258-0659-1

© 2024 by the authors. Articles in this book are Open Access and distributed under the Creative Commons Attribution (CC BY) license. The book as a whole is distributed by MDPI under the terms and conditions of the Creative Commons Attribution-NonCommercial-NoDerivs (CC BY-NC-ND) license.

# Contents

About the Editor . . . . . . . . . . . . . . . . . . . . . . . . . . . . . . . . . . . . . . . . . . vii

**Frauke Wilken, Peter Buschner, Christian Benignus, Anna-Maria Behr, Johannes Rieger and Johannes Beckmann**
Pharmatherapeutic Treatment of Osteoarthrosis—Does the Pill against Already Exist? A Narrative Review
Reprinted from: *J. Pers. Med.* 2023, 13, 1087, doi:10.3390/jpm13071087 . . . . . . . . . . . . . . . 1

**Anand S. Dhaliwal, Muzammil Akhtar, Daniel I. Razick, Arya Afzali, Ethan Wilson and Alexander J. Nedopil**
Current Surgical Techniques in the Treatment of Adult Developmental Dysplasia of the Hip
Reprinted from: *J. Pers. Med.* 2023, 13, 942, doi:10.3390/jpm13060942 . . . . . . . . . . . . . . . 13

**Sébastien Parratte, Jeremy Daxhelet, Jean-Noel Argenson and Cécile Batailler**
The Deep-MCL Line: A Reliable Anatomical Landmark to Optimize the Tibial Cut in UKA
Reprinted from: *J. Pers. Med.* 2023, 13, 855, doi:10.3390/jpm13050855 . . . . . . . . . . . . . . . 32

**Julien Lebleu, Andries Pauwels, Philippe Anract, Sébastien Parratte, Philippe Van Overschelde and Stefaan Van Onsem**
Digital Rehabilitation after Knee Arthroplasty: A Multi-Center Prospective Longitudinal Cohort Study
Reprinted from: *J. Pers. Med.* 2023, 13, 824, doi:10.3390/jpm13050824 . . . . . . . . . . . . . . . 42

**James W. Pritchett**
Cementless Metal-Free Ceramic-Coated Shoulder Resurfacing
Reprinted from: *J. Pers. Med.* 2023, 13, 825, doi:10.3390/jpm13050825 . . . . . . . . . . . . . . . 53

**Dominik Rak, Lukas Klann, Tizian Heinz, Philip Anderson, Ioannis Stratos and Alexander J. Nedopil et al.**
Influence of Mechanical Alignment on Functional Knee Phenotypes and Clinical Outcomes in Primary TKA: A 1-Year Prospective Analysis
Reprinted from: *J. Pers. Med.* 2023, 13, 778, doi:10.3390/jpm13050778 . . . . . . . . . . . . . . . 63

**Patrick Weber, Melina Beck, Michael Klug, Andreas Klug, Alexander Klug and Claudio Glowalla et al.**
Survival of Patient-Specific Unicondylar Knee Replacement
Reprinted from: *J. Pers. Med.* 2023, 13, 665, doi:10.3390/jpm13040665 . . . . . . . . . . . . . . . 73

**Christian Benignus, Peter Buschner, Malin Kristin Meier, Frauke Wilken, Johannes Rieger and Johannes Beckmann**
Patient Specific Instruments and Patient Individual Implants—A Narrative Review
Reprinted from: *J. Pers. Med.* 2023, 13, 426, doi:10.3390/jpm13030426 . . . . . . . . . . . . . . . 85

**Lieke Sweerts, Pepijn W. Dekkers, Philip J. van der Wees, Job L. C. van Susante, Lex D. de Jong and Thomas J. Hoogeboom et al.**
External Validation of Prediction Models for Surgical Complications in People Considering Total Hip or Knee Arthroplasty Was Successful for Delirium but Not for Surgical Site Infection, Postoperative Bleeding, and Nerve Damage: A Retrospective Cohort Study
Reprinted from: *J. Pers. Med.* 2023, 13, 277, doi:10.3390/jpm13020277 . . . . . . . . . . . . . . . 96

**Adrian C. Ruckli, Andreas K. Nanavati, Malin K. Meier, Till D. Lerch, Simon D. Steppacher and Sébastian Vuilleumier et al.**
A Deep Learning Method for Quantification of Femoral Head Necrosis Based on Routine Hip MRI for Improved Surgical Decision Making
Reprinted from: *J. Pers. Med.* **2023**, *13*, 153, doi:10.3390/jpm13010153 . . . . . . . . . . . . . . . . **106**

**Johannes Beckmann, David Barrett and Emmanuel Thienpont**
Cutting-Edge Approaches in Arthroplasty: Before, during and after Surgery
Reprinted from: *J. Pers. Med.* **2022**, *12*, 1671, doi:10.3390/jpm12101671 . . . . . . . . . . . . . . . . **118**

# About the Editor

**Johannes Beckmann**

Prof. Dr. Johannes Beckmann is the Chief Doctor at the Orthopedics and Accident Surgery Clinic, where he has 130 beds and performs thousands of operations every year, including thousands of artificial joints of the knees and hips.

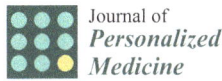

Review

# Pharmatherapeutic Treatment of Osteoarthrosis—Does the Pill against Already Exist? A Narrative Review

Frauke Wilken [1,*], Peter Buschner [1], Christian Benignus [2], Anna-Maria Behr [1], Johannes Rieger [1] and Johannes Beckmann [1]

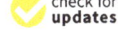

Citation: Wilken, F.; Buschner, P.; Benignus, C.; Behr, A.-M.; Rieger, J.; Beckmann, J. Pharmatherapeutic Treatment of Osteoarthrosis—Does the Pill against Already Exist? A Narrative Review. *J. Pers. Med.* **2023**, *13*, 1087. https://doi.org/10.3390/jpm13071087

Academic Editor: Peter Pilot

Received: 12 June 2023
Revised: 23 June 2023
Accepted: 26 June 2023
Published: 30 June 2023

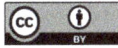

**Copyright:** © 2023 by the authors. Licensee MDPI, Basel, Switzerland. This article is an open access article distributed under the terms and conditions of the Creative Commons Attribution (CC BY) license (https://creativecommons.org/licenses/by/4.0/).

[1] Department of Orthopedic Surgery and Traumatology, Hospital Barmherzige Brüder Munich, Romanstr. 93, 80639 München, Germany; peter.buschner@barmherzige-muenchen.de (P.B.); anna-maria.behr@barmherzige-muenchen.de (A.-M.B.); johannes.rieger2@barmherzige-muenchen.de (J.R.); johannes.beckmann@barmherzige-muenchen.de (J.B.)

[2] Department of Traumatology and Orthopedic Surgery, Hospital Ludwigsburg, Posilipostr. 4, 71640 Ludwigsburg, Germany; christian.benignus@rkh-gesundheit.de

* Correspondence: frauke.wilken@barmherzige-muenchen.de

**Abstract:** The aim of this narrative review is to summarize the current pharmacotherapeutic treatment options for osteoarthritis (OA). Is therapy still mainly symptomatic or does the pill against arthrosis already exist? Causal and non-causal, as well as future therapeutic approaches, are discussed. Various surgical and non-surgical treatment options are available that can help manage symptoms, slow down progression, and improve quality of life. To date, however, therapy is still mainly symptomatic, often using painkilling and anti-inflammatory drugs until the final stage, which is usually joint replacement. These "symptomatic pills against" have side effects and do not alter the progression of OA, which is caused by an imbalance between degenerative and regenerative processes. Next to resolving mechanical issues, the goal must be to gain a better understanding of the cellular and molecular basis of OA. Recently, there has been a lot of interest in cartilage-regenerative medicine and in the current style of treating rheumatoid arthritis, where drug therapy ("the pill against") has been established to slow down or even stop the progression of rheumatoid arthritis and has banned the vast majority of former almost regular severe joint destructions. However, the "causal pill against" OA does not exist so far. First, the early detection of osteoarthritis by means of biomarkers and imaging should therefore gain more focus. Second, future therapeutic approaches have to identify innovative therapeutic approaches influencing inflammatory and metabolic processes. Several pharmacologic, genetic, and even epigenetic attempts are promising, but none have clinically improved causal therapy so far, unfortunately.

**Keywords:** osteoarthritis; cartilage; chondroprotectors; platelet rich plasma; NSAIDs; mesenchymal stem cells

## 1. Introduction

Osteoarthritis (OA) is a disease with a degenerative and inflammatory component that affects a large proportion of the ageing population [1]. The joints of the lower extremities are particularly affected, especially the hip and knee. Cartilage loss is the most visible change, but all joint structures are affected, some occurring quite a bit earlier than cartilage, such as the synovia or subchondral bone. OA involves a variety of factors, such as mechanical loading, ageing, inflammation, and metabolic changes, and the activation of different signaling pathways and enzymatic processes, ultimately leading to a progressive loss of joint function. Consequently, osteoarthritis is a heterogeneous disease with a common end route but many different starting points. Accordingly, there are diverse treatment modalities. They can either be conservative such as thermal, pharmacological, orthotic or physiotherapeutic, or surgical. The latter can be reconstructive, such as in cartilage stimulation or cartilage transplantation, load allocating, such as in osteotomies, or finally replacing, such as in terms of artificial joint replacement. However, especially in the early stages, the therapeutic approach often remains purely symptomatic. Currently, there is no causal drug for the treatment of OA. The most common treatment form is the use of painkilling and anti-inflammatory drugs until the final stage of treatment, which is usually joint replacement. However, the actual cause of OA is often not being treated. Another recent narrative review summarized the guidelines and symptomatic pharmacotherapeutic treatments [2].

The current review's aim is to describe future perspectives. In recent years, the pathogenesis of osteoarthritis has become increasingly well understood, and new therapeutic approaches are emerging. There are clear similarities to rheumatoid arthritis, which led to a large number of rapid and severe joint destructions several decades ago. Today, those cases are rare due to new medical approaches, mainly the so-called biologicals [3]. The goal is to implement causal therapy and to abandon singular symptomatic therapy in OA as well. By influencing the underlying signaling pathways of OA or by using stem cells, attempts have been made to prevent the destruction of cartilage or to reduce the pain-triggering inflammatory reaction. The development of OA pharmacotherapies is primarily focused on the protection or even the regeneration of cartilage tissue, led by the assumption that the protection of cartilage structure also influences the clinical symptoms. Contradictorily, an MRI-based study has shown that a loss of cartilage thickness is associated with only a small amount of worsening knee pain, an association mediated in part by worsening synovitis [4]. Possible therapeutic approaches are, therefore, in addition to chondroprotection, the causal treatment of synovitis.

The aim of this narrative review is to summarize the current pharmacotherapeutic treatment options for OA therapy beyond the solely symptomatic attempts. Causal and non-causal, as well as future, therapeutic approaches are discussed below. This review attempts to think outside the box by also mentioning the approaches in the field of gene therapy and epigenetics. OA therapies that are not drug therapies are not addressed in this review. Lifestyle modifications, such as a change in eating habits and dietary weight management, as well as activity, physiotherapy, and mechanical issues also play a large part in successful therapy. A claim to the completeness of all possible therapy alternatives for OA can therefore not be made. The question addressed here is whether OA therapy will remain mainly symptomatic or if the pill against arthrosis already exists?

## 2. Symptomatic OA Therapy

*2.1. Pain Killers*

The most common therapy for OA is still the use of painkillers. In principle, there are different classes of substances available. These drugs are a purely symptomatic therapy that can alleviate but cannot influence the progression of OA. As this topic has been well described in several guidelines and in a recent narrative review [2], just a short summary of the most used painkillers will be presented in the following.

Nonsteroidal anti-inflammatory drugs (NSAIDs) are the most commonly used and prescribed pain medications in the treatment of OA and are routinely recommended in clinical practice guidelines [5]. Pain management is an essential part of OA treatment. Inflammation occurs in all joint tissues and is thus an essential target of drug therapy. Inflammation leads to the release of various neuromodulatory mediators such as cytokines and prostaglandins which are synthesized by the enzyme cyclooxygenase (COX). The release of proinflammatory mediators leads to the classic symptoms of synovitis, joint swelling and hyperthermia. Furthermore, inflammation can induce joint tissue damage [6–8].

NSAIDs can counteract these processes by reducing the corresponding inflammatory cascades by inhibiting the COX enzyme. Additionally, NSAIDs can reduce the sensation of pain relief by desensitizing nociceptors and are thus effective drugs in the symptomatic therapy of OA [9]. Smith et al. and Stewart et al. report in their meta-analysis that oral NSAIDs are similarly effective as opioids in relieving pain in patients with OA [10,11].

However, the use of NSAIDS is limited due to their known but rare risk of gastrointestinal, cardiovascular, and renal adverse events [12].

Studies have concluded that the oral use of NSAIDs is mainly recommended for short-term or intermittent therapy, rather than prolonged treatment [13]. Osani et al. reported in their meta-analysis that the therapeutic peak of NSAID-induced benefits in patients with knee OA was reached after 2 weeks and decreased over time, while cardiovascular and gastrointestinal side effects were already significantly increased after 4 weeks of treatment.

The usage of selective COX-2 inhibitors has increased in the past decades, due to their benefit of combining both anti-inflammatory and analgesic properties, while providing better gastrointestinal tolerability and a reduction in gastroduodenal ulcers in comparison with non-selective COX inhibitors [14].

Coxibs, however, have been associated with an increase in cardiovascular events due to a reduction in prostaglandin synthesis [15]. On the contrary, in a meta-analysis conducted by Cooper et al., recent data has shown that celecoxib does not significantly increase cardiovascular risk when compared with conventional NSAIDs and placebos, regardless of the dose and the duration of treatment [16]. However, recommendations on the analgesic use of various NSAIDs for patients with underlying health conditions remain conflicting. When prescribing any type of NSAIDs, all risk factors (age, gastrointestinal, cardiovascular, and renal events) should be taken into account. Due to adverse effects, NSAIDs are not intended for long term treatment.

A simple and effective way to reduce the risk of gastrointestinal side effects is the topical application of NSAIDs. Amemiya et al. compared the effects of esflurbiprofen patches versus flurbiprofen tablets in patients with gonarthrosis in 2021. Maximum esflurbiprofen concentrations were observed in the synovium, synovial fluids, and plasma after esflurbiprofen plaster (SFPP) application for 12 h. The numeric rating scale (NRS) results indicated a long-lasting effect of SFPP. Through transdermal application, a continuously high drug effect level was achieved. Overall, no dose peaks need to be accepted to achieve the same effect as with repeated daily oral administration [17].

Depending on the risk profile and the patient's pain perception, it must be decided on a case-by-case basis whether oral or topical application is preferable.

Opioids are an alternative for more severe pain states when usual pain medication or other pain treatments are not sufficient or may not be used. In a direct comparison with NSAIDs, tramadol was inferior in terms of analgesia [18]. When prescribing opioids, the side effect profile, such as central nervous effects with fatigue, dizziness, and impaired balance, should be taken into account. This is where opioids differ adversely from NSAIDs. Opioids such as tramadol should not be prescribed as a first-line therapy. If other drugs are not used due to their side effect profile or if a non-drug therapy (e.g., surgery) is not currently available, they should be used. Opioids are not used long-term or routinely for osteoarthritis. However, they may be indicated for short-term therapy [2].

*2.2. Symptomatic OA Therapy with Potentially Causal Impact*

2.2.1. Hyaluronic Acid (Intra-Articular)

Hyaluronic acid (HA) is reduced in both concentration and molecular size in patients with osteoarthritis; hence, the intra-articular injection of HA aims to substitute the physiological synovial HA. The individual hyaluronic acid (HA) products differ in terms of production, molecular weight, degree of cross-linking, viscosity, and frequency of application per series. Despite a large number of scientific studies, the effectiveness of this therapy is still disputed in the literature. While some meta-analyses show tangible benefits, they often include studies with a high risk of bias. When meta-analyses are restricted to studies with a low risk of bias, the effect of IAHA is similar to that of saline injections [2,19]. There is a growing amount of literature demonstrating that product differences, particularly HA molecular weight, may have a significant effect on treatment outcomes, with a higher molecular weight showing better results [19]. Due to the invasive mode of application, the indication for intra-articular HA injection should, however, only be made when the prescription of NSAIDs is not possible due to side effects or contraindications or when these are not sufficiently effective. The possible side effects such as joint infection or irritation of the knee joint must be discussed with the patient in advance; severe adverse events are rare.

### 2.2.2. Corticosteroids (Intra-Articular)

The intra-articular injection of a glucocorticoid for the relief of the acute inflammatory symptoms of activated arthrosis can be a useful measure. The aim of the treatment is to reduce pain and restore mobility. Randomised and placebo-controlled studies have shown that the intra-articular injection of a glucocorticoid into an osteoarthritic knee joint can significantly reduce symptoms over a period of at least 1 week. Occasionally, however, a prolonged effect lasting 16–24 weeks is observed after the intra-articular application of glucocorticoids [20]. They should be used in the short term at the lowest possible but effective dosage for painful arthrosis that does not respond to other therapeutic measures. This may be the case, for example, in inflamed arthrosis with acute pain exacerbation.

There is a lack of data on the long-term effects of cortisone injections on articular cartilage and on a possible association with adverse joint effects. However, in some in vivo studies, corticosteroids were found to be cytotoxic to articular cartilage [21]. In a 2-year randomised trial, the cortisone-infiltration group showed higher cartilage loss than the saline-injection group. Taken together, cortisone injections are still a common treatment option, but they are not without side effects. Frequent use must therefore be considered critically [22]. Injections at too short intervals increase the risk of infection. The patient should be informed about the possible complications of infection and/or tissue atrophy as well as about possible treatment alternatives.

### 2.2.3. Platelet-Rich Plasma (Intra-Articular)

Aside from the available oral drugs against OA, the usage of autologous growth factors, e.g., intra-articular injections of platelet-rich plasma (PRP), can be used for OA treatment, especially for knee OA. The autologous fluid, which is obtained by centrifuging whole blood, is a highly concentrated cocktail of inflammatory mediators and growth factors capable of reducing inflammatory distress and stimulating cell proliferation and cartilaginous matrix production [16]. Between 2011 and 2021, 867 studies on the topic of PRP were published, with an upward trend over the years [23].

Multiple studies have confirmed effective pain relief and the improvement of physical function after PRP injections as well as an acceptable safety profile [24,25].

PRP injections also showed stronger effects compared with conventional injections with corticosteroids and hyaluronic acid [24]. Furthermore, regular injections of intra-articular corticosteroid can lead to the loss of cartilage structure and thus more rapid disease progression.

Consequently, PRP injections may not only contribute to pain relief through anti-inflammatory effects but can also provide lasting pain relief and functional restoration through targeted structural reconstruction when used over an extended period of time.

It was shown that PRP injections significantly improved physical function and WOMAC scores at 3, and up to 12, months [24].

Patients undergoing treatment with PRP injections experience both pain relief and improved joint function. However, it remains unclear whether the short-term effect of PRP injection is due to the temporary changes in the joint environment or whether PRP injections actually lead to structural changes, thus preventing the progression of OA. Another unresolved question surrounds which components of PRP cause this effect. In particular, the proportion of leukocytes (leukocyte-rich or leukocyte-poor) is still the subject of research. The first positive results have been achieved with leukocyte-poor plasma [26]. In summary, the use of PRP is showing very encouraging preliminary results; however, its use is not yet recommended as first-line-therapy in the guidelines.

### 2.2.4. Chondroitin and Glucosamine

Chondroitin and glucosamine have chondroprotective, analgesic, and anti-inflammatory effects. They are symptomatic, slow-acting drugs used against osteoarthritis. Glucosamine is a component of glycosaminoglycans and can be found in high amounts in articular cartilage and synovial fluid. Chondroitin is found in the extracellular matrix of articular cartilage and plays a role in maintaining osmotic pressure. Thus, it could improve elasticity and the resistance of cartilage [27]. Both chondroitin and glucosamine seem to develop their effects—partly in different forms—through the use of many different pathways. However, only a few selected ones will be mentioned below. Glucosamine was shown to decrease the levels of proinflammatory interleukin-1 (IL-1), interleukin-6 (IL-6), tumor necrosis factor-$\alpha$ (TNF-$\alpha$), and C-reactive protein (CRP) in studies with rats. In contrast, the anti-inflammatory interleukins IL-2 and IL-10 were increased [28–30]. Glucosamine also appears to have immunomodulatory effects that affect the activity of phospholipase A2, matrix metalloproteinases, or aggrecans [31]. Moreover, chondroitin and glucosamine block the pathways involved in inflammation in osteoarthritis, such as the mitogen-activated protein kinase (MAPK) pathway [32]. In addition, both chondroitin and glucosamine have antioxidant effects [33].

In a meta-analysis by Zhu et al. from 2018, it was shown that chondroitin—via oral administration—significantly alleviates pain and leads to an improvement in physical function compared with a placebo. Glucosamine, on the other hand, may improve stiffness [34]. A combination of glucosamine and chondroitin appears to provide better pain relief than acetaminophen in hip and knee OA, but celecoxib showed the best results in this study [35]. It was found that both chondroitin alone and glucosamine alone could significantly reduce the decrease in joint space. Moreover, intraarticular injections of hyaluronic acid in combination with glucosamine hydrochloride led to a significantly higher reduction in IL-6, IL-1$\beta$, and TGF-$\beta$ compared with hyaluronic acid alone in patients with temporomandibular OA [36].

Kwoh et al. and Fransen et al. failed to demonstrate any changes in joint structure with chondroitin or glucosamine administration in patients with chronic knee pain in OA [37,38]. Another meta-analysis summarized seventeen studies, of which only seven studies demonstrated a statistically significant reduction in pain and four studies demonstrated a reduction in joint space narrowing [39].

Several smaller dosages of glucosamine throughout the day appear to be more effective than one large dose per day [40].

Taken together, chondroitin and glucosamine seem to have an effect on the milder forms of OA, reducing joint inflammation and pain. The administration is safe and shows only a small number of adverse effects, such as headache or nausea. Overall, however, there are conflicting results regarding their clinical efficacy. Thus, in patients with contraindications to NSAIDs or with an increased risk of gastrointestinal or cardiovascular risks, the use of oral glucosamine and chondroitin may be considered as a treatment trial before more invasive therapies are undertaken.

### 2.2.5. Collagen

Collagen is a protein of the extracellular matrix that occurs mainly as collagen type II in the articular cartilage. The enteral absorption of undenatured type II collagen is very low, but di- or tripeptides containing the amino acids proline or hydroxyproline can be absorbed and show an effect [41]. Hydrolyzed collagen could contribute to cartilage regeneration by increasing the synthesis of macromolecules in the extracellular matrix [42]. In addition, collagen is able to modulate both humoral and cellular components of the immune system. It contributes to the body's ability to distinguish between harmless molecules and potentially harmful pathogens [43]. This leads, for example, to the transformation of naive T cells into T regulatory cells that produce anti-inflammatory substances such as TGF-$\beta$ and IL-10 [44]. Proline and hydroxyproline can induce hyaluronic acid synthesis [45] and the chondrocytes to synthesize glycosaminoglycans [46].

Pain in patients with hip and knee OA can be alleviated using an oral supplementation of collagen. WOMAC scores, VAS scores, and quality of life improve significantly compared with a placebo [47]. Trc et al. compared a supplementation of hydrolyzed collagen and glucosamine sulphate for 90 days, respectively. The supplementation of hydrolyzed collagen led to a statistically significant improvement in WOMAC and VAS scores compared with glucosamine sulphate [48].

Joint conditions seem to improve following the administration of collagen. It may induce cartilage repair to maintain structure and function. The clinical use of collagen is safe and has minimal adverse effects, mainly gastrointestinal. However, further studies are needed to show the benefits in the treatment of patients with OA and to determine the optimal dosage and duration.

## 3. Causal OA Therapy

### 3.1. Monoclonal Antibodies

Over the last few decades, monoclonal antibodies have emerged as a revolutionary tool in the field of medicine with many promising clinical applications. One of the biggest advantages of monoclonal antibodies is their high specificity as they are designed to target molecules in the body such as cytokines, growth factors, and receptors. In the context of osteoarthritis, antibodies revolutionized the treatment of rheumatoid arthritis. Currently, drug therapy ("the pill against") has been established to slow down or even stop the progression of the autoimmune disease and has caused the end of the vast majority of formerly regular severe joint destructions. Although the effects and goals of treatment are partly comparable to OA, they are not established as standard therapy. The question arises, will this change? Up to now, there have been some approaches that use monoclonal antibodies in pain therapy of OA, some of which will be presented in the following.

#### 3.1.1. TNF and IL-1 Inhibitors

In one randomized controlled trial, patients with erosive hand OA were treated with the anti-TNF antibody adalimumab (subcutaneous administration once a week) or a placebo for 12 weeks each. Pain intensity was measured with the VAS score. There was no significant difference [49]. Another anti-TNF antibody (etanercept) failed to demonstrate any benefit in a treatment duration of 24 weeks compared with a placebo in hand OA [50]. Canakinumab is an IL-1 inhibitor that showed a reduced rate of joint arthroplasties in patients with atherosclerotic disease [51]. However, further studies failed to show any benefits with respect to pain alleviation in patients with OA when IL-1 was blocked [52]. Overall, TNF and IL-1 inhibitors seem to be rather unsuitable for patients with OA.

#### 3.1.2. Anti-NGF

Joint tissues have been innervated using nociceptors, except for cartilage. Nerve growth factor is an important neurotrophin in inflamed synovium. It is upregulated in patients with OA and leads to an increase in pain. There are three different monoclonal antibodies used in therapy: Tanezumab, Ulranumab, and Fasinumab. They lead to impressive pain relief in patients with knee and hip OA but accelerate the progression of OA [53]. The administration of fewer doses showed a reduced but still substantial effect on pain and function. Nevertheless, 3% of the patients suffered from progressive OA [54]. There are a few other adverse effects such as peripheral neuropathies, headaches, upper respiratory tract infections, oedema, or joint pain [55]. NGF seems to be a relevant factor for cartilage integrity or the repair of cartilage, so that a complete blockade is not an effective treatment in patients with OA. Anti-NGF treatment is promising, but studies are needed to find the optimal dosage to alleviate pain and reduce the adverse effects.

### 3.2. Stem Cell Treatments

Mesenchymal stem cells (MSCs), as a specific type of adult stem cell, possess great potential in regenerative therapy due to their capacity for self-renewal and differentiation [56]. Great attention has been paid to cell-based therapy that may influence cartilage repair such as mesenchymal stem cell therapy. Most studies have been conducted in the context of knee joint osteoarthritis. MSCs are primarily used as intra-articular injection therapy. MSCs modulate immune or inflammatory effects and tissue regeneration in knee osteoarthritis [57,58]. The exact mechanism of MSC therapy remains unclear. It is known that cartilage repair and protection against OA-induced cartilage degeneration is promoted by MSC-derived extracellular vesicles.

Injected MSCs are expected to repair damaged issues due to the trilineage potential and immunomodulatory properties of MSCs. MSCs can be harvested from different sites. The best known or most accessible sites are bone marrow or fat tissue. Other sources include muscle tissue, synovial membranes, or placenta. In addition, the cells can be obtained either from autogenic or allogenic sources. The advantage of allogenic stem cells is that they can be harvested from healthy donors and expanded in vitro to obtain a clinically relevant amount for injection. The disadvantage of allogeneic cell collection is a possible reaction of the recipient's immune system after injection [59].

Studies in humans have reported variable structural outcomes after MSC injection from hyaline-like cartilage to fibrous tissue. A meta-analysis including 582 knee-OA-patients in 11 trials was performed to assess the efficacy and safety of MSC treatment for knee OA patients using VAS, IKDC, WOMAC, Lequesne, Lysholm, and Tegner scores. MSC-treatment groups from the identified trials were compared with their respective control groups. It shows that VAS decreases and IKDC increases significantly after 24 months follow up. MSC therapy also showed significant decreases in WOMAC and Lequesne scores after the 12-month follow up. The evaluation of Lysholm (24-month) and Tegner (12- and 24-month) scores also demonstrated favorable results for MSC treatment. The effects of MSC therapy on short-term primary endpoints still need to be evaluated in a larger number of patients [60].

Another important question is the dosage at which the stem cells should be injected. A larger amount of injected MSCs may be expected to induce better effects. Interestingly, in studies with allogeneic stem cells, it was found that no improvement was observed in relation to "high dose" as opposed to "low dose" stem cell transplantation. The clinical symptoms and MRI imaging of the cartilage were the main factors assessed. There were also differences in the dose effect of stem cells depending on their origin. These results suggest that appropriate MSC doses applied in intra-articular injections to OA patients need to be determined for each origin of MSCs [61,62]. Furthermore, MSC injection combined with other agents such as hyaluronic acid [63] or PRP [64] has better therapeutic effects than MSC injection alone. This implies the possible value of drug cocktail therapy when using MSC injection in knee OA patients.

Overall, MSC transplantation treatment was shown to be safe and has great potential as an efficacious clinical therapy, especially for patients with knee OA. Further clinical and in vitro studies are needed to better clarify the underlying molecular and biochemical mechanisms. Particularly, it is yet to be determined whether MSCs should be injected as a single agent or in combination with another drug or as a complementary therapy to surgical treatment.

## 4. Future Directions

### 4.1. Gene Therapy

Gene therapy consists of using a vector to bring genes directly into cells and tissues to treat a specific disease. Viral vectors include RNA viruses and DNA viruses. Two different gene therapy strategies are currently in preclinical and clinical development for OA [65]. The first approach consists of ex vivo modifying and amplifying cells, followed by their intra-articular injection. The aim is to over-express TGF-ß-1 in irradiated allogenic chondrocytes [66]. The second approach is an in vivo gene therapy through the local or systemic injection of viral vectors containing the transgene of interest. In general, OA gene therapy aims to reduce inflammation through overexpressing transgenes such as IL-1Ra or a soluble TNF receptor [67]. In the future, gene therapy could become a strategy to regulate the intra-articular expression of therapeutic targets in OA.

*4.2. Epigenetics*

Epigenetics is a field of research that analyzes the changes in gene expression or cell phenotype occurring without the modification of the DNA sequence. Several epigenetic regulators appear to be involved in the pathogenesis of OA. The epigenetic profiling of articular chondrocytes has revealed the existence of an activating sequence that is present in billions of people with a risk locus (GDF5-UQCC1) that is involved in OA progression. These epigenetic modifications can also suppress the expression of protective genes in OA [61]. Abnormal changes in DNA methylation occur in the promoter regions of related genes and signaling pathways in OA chondrocytes. Epigenetic regulation typically involves DNA methylation, histone modification, and noncoding RNA-mediated regulation. Epigenetic mechanisms can control several signaling pathways simultaneously. For this reason, epigenetic modifications have been considered a potential therapeutic target to manage OA [68].

## 5. Conclusions

OA is caused by an imbalance between degenerative and regenerative processes. To date, therapy is still mainly symptomatic. As well as improving mechanical issues, the future therapeutic goal must be to gain an even better understanding of the cellular and molecular causes of OA. Non-surgical therapy comprises basic measures such as weight reduction, exercise therapy (water and land), and health education. Specific measures comprise biomechanical interventions, physiotherapy, physical measures, and drug therapy. Several pharmacologic, genetic, and even epigenetic attempts are promising, but unfortunately, so far none have proven causal therapy to work or cure OA. The early detection of osteoarthritis by means of biomarkers and imaging must also gain focus to allow for early and targeted treatment.

With regards to drug therapy, the individual risk profile as well as the level of suffering or pain intensity must be taken into account before treatment is started. For this reason, it is not possible to give general advice on drug therapy for OA. A non-causal but proven treatment option for OA is the use of painkillers (mainly NSAIDs), which are beyond the focus of this review. Their duration of therapy is limited due to side effects, especially in patients with corresponding underlying diseases. They are solely symptomatic, therefore alleviate but do not alter the progression of OA. The use of PRP injections seems to clearly overcome hyaluronic acid which has recently shown conflicting results. PRP can potentially stimulate cell proliferation and cartilaginous matrix production and provide lasting pain relief and functional restoration through targeted structural reconstruction when used over an extended period of time. Therapies with chondroprotective substances such as chondroitin, glucosamine, collagen, or monoclonal antibodies lead to a reduction in pain. However, a significant therapeutic effect in singular application has not been detected so far. The use of stem cells in arthrosis therapy, however, is a promising therapy. Its possibility for cell regeneration or conversion into functional cells holds great potential, especially in the context of the therapy of degenerative diseases such as OA. Favored cell sources, dosage, and therapy duration remain unclear.

Due to the multifactorial genesis of OA, most therapeutic approaches are still symptomatic and the "causal pill against" OA does not yet exist. Future therapeutic approaches have to identify innovative therapeutic targets aimed at influencing the inflammatory and metabolic processes underlying the pathogenesis and progression of OA.

**Author Contributions:** Conceptualization, J.B. and F.W.; methodology, J.B. and F.W.; software, F.W.; validation, J.B. and F.W.; formal analysis, J.B. and F.W.; investigation, J.B. and F.W.; resources, J.B. and F.W.; data curation, F.W.; writing—original draft preparation, F.W., P.B., A.-M.B., and C.B.; writing—review and editing, J.B. and F.W.; visualization, J.R.; supervision, J.B. and F.W.; project administration,

J.B. and F.W.; funding acquisition, J.B. All authors have read and agreed to the published version of the manuscript.

**Funding:** This research received no external funding.

**Institutional Review Board Statement:** Not applicable.

**Informed Consent Statement:** Not applicable.

**Data Availability Statement:** Not applicable.

**Conflicts of Interest:** The authors declare no conflict of interest.

## References

1. Das, S.K.; Farooqi, A. Osteoarthritis. *Best Pract. Res. Clin. Rheumatol.* **2008**, *22*, 657–675. [CrossRef]
2. Richard, M.J.; Driban, J.B.; McAlindon, T.E. Pharmaceutical treatment of osteoarthritis. *Osteoarthr. Cartil.* **2023**, *31*, 458–466. [CrossRef] [PubMed]
3. Smolen, J.S.; Landewe, R.B.M.; Bijlsma, J.W.J.; Burmester, G.R.; Dougados, M.; Kerschbaumer, A.; McInnes, I.B.; Sepriano, A.; van Vollenhoven, R.F.; de Wit, M.; et al. EULAR recommendations for the management of rheumatoid arthritis with synthetic and biological disease-modifying antirheumatic drugs: 2019 update. *Ann. Rheum. Dis.* **2020**, *79*, 685–699. [CrossRef] [PubMed]
4. Bacon, K.; LaValley, M.P.; Jafarzadeh, S.R.; Felson, D. Does cartilage loss cause pain in osteoarthritis and if so, how much? *Ann. Rheum. Dis.* **2020**, *79*, 1105–1110. [CrossRef]
5. Arden, N.K.; Perry, T.A.; Bannuru, R.R.; Bruyere, O.; Cooper, C.; Haugen, I.K.; Hochberg, M.C.; McAlindon, T.E.; Mobasheri, A.; Reginster, J.Y. Non-surgical management of knee osteoarthritis: Comparison of ESCEO and OARSI 2019 guidelines. *Nat. Rev. Rheumatol.* **2021**, *17*, 59–66. [CrossRef]
6. Dawes, J.M.; Kiesewetter, H.; Perkins, J.R.; Bennett, D.L.; McMahon, S.B. Chemokine expression in peripheral tissues from the monosodium iodoacetate model of chronic joint pain. *Mol. Pain* **2013**, *9*, 57. [CrossRef] [PubMed]
7. Driscoll, C.; Chanalaris, A.; Knights, C.; Ismail, H.; Sacitharan, P.K.; Gentry, C.; Bevan, S.; Vincent, T.L. Nociceptive Sensitizers Are Regulated in Damaged Joint Tissues, Including Articular Cartilage, When Osteoarthritic Mice Display Pain Behavior. *Arthritis Rheumatol.* **2016**, *68*, 857–867. [CrossRef]
8. Pinho-Ribeiro, F.A.; Verri, W.A., Jr.; Chiu, I.M. Nociceptor Sensory Neuron-Immune Interactions in Pain and Inflammation. *Trends Immunol.* **2017**, *38*, 5–19. [CrossRef]
9. Osani, M.C.; Vaysbrot, E.E.; Zhou, M.; McAlindon, T.E.; Bannuru, R.R. Duration of Symptom Relief and Early Trajectory of Adverse Events for Oral Nonsteroidal Antiinflammatory Drugs in Knee Osteoarthritis: A Systematic Review and Meta-Analysis. *Arthritis Care Res.* **2020**, *72*, 641–651. [CrossRef]
10. Smith, S.R.; Deshpande, B.R.; Collins, J.E.; Katz, J.N.; Losina, E. Comparative pain reduction of oral non-steroidal anti-inflammatory drugs and opioids for knee osteoarthritis: Systematic analytic review. *Osteoarthr. Cartil.* **2016**, *24*, 962–972. [CrossRef] [PubMed]
11. Stewart, M.; Cibere, J.; Sayre, E.C.; Kopec, J.A. Efficacy of commonly prescribed analgesics in the management of osteoarthritis: A systematic review and meta-analysis. *Rheumatol. Int.* **2018**, *38*, 1985–1997. [CrossRef] [PubMed]
12. O'Neil, C.K.; Hanlon, J.T.; Marcum, Z.A. Adverse effects of analgesics commonly used by older adults with osteoarthritis: Focus on non-opioid and opioid analgesics. *Am. J. Geriatr. Pharmacother.* **2012**, *10*, 331–342. [CrossRef] [PubMed]
13. Bannuru, R.R.; Osani, M.C.; Vaysbrot, E.E.; Arden, N.K.; Bennell, K.; Bierma-Zeinstra, S.M.A.; Kraus, V.B.; Lohmander, L.S.; Abbott, J.H.; Bhandari, M.; et al. OARSI guidelines for the non-surgical management of knee, hip, and polyarticular osteoarthritis. *Osteoarthr. Cartil.* **2019**, *27*, 1578–1589. [CrossRef] [PubMed]
14. Coxib and Traditional NSAID Trialists' (CNT) Collaboration; Bhala, N.; Emberson, J.; Merhi, A.; Abramson, S.; Arber, N.; Baron, J.A.; Bombardier, C.; Cannon, C.; Farkouh, M.E.; et al. Vascular and upper gastrointestinal effects of non-steroidal anti-inflammatory drugs: Meta-analyses of individual participant data from randomised trials. *Lancet* **2013**, *382*, 769–779. [CrossRef]
15. Gunter, B.R.; Butler, K.A.; Wallace, R.L.; Smith, S.M.; Harirforoosh, S. Non-steroidal anti-inflammatory drug-induced cardiovascular adverse events: A meta-analysis. *J. Clin. Pharm. Ther.* **2017**, *42*, 27–38. [CrossRef]
16. Cooper, D.L.; Harirforoosh, S. Effect of formulation variables on preparation of celecoxib loaded polylactide-co-glycolide nanoparticles. *PLoS ONE* **2014**, *9*, e113558. [CrossRef]
17. Amemiya, M.; Nakagawa, Y.; Yoshimura, H.; Takahashi, T.; Inomata, K.; Nagase, T.; Ju, Y.J.; Shimaya, M.; Tsukada, S.; Hirasawa, N.; et al. Comparison of tissue pharmacokinetics of esflurbiprofen plaster with flurbiprofen tablets in patients with knee osteoarthritis: A multicenter randomized controlled trial. *Biopharm. Drug Dispos.* **2021**, *42*, 418–426. [CrossRef] [PubMed]
18. Welsch, P.; Sommer, C.; Schiltenwolf, M.; Hauser, W. Opioids in chronic noncancer pain-are opioids superior to nonopioid analgesics? A systematic review and meta-analysis of efficacy, tolerability and safety in randomized head-to-head comparisons of opioids versus nonopioid analgesics of at least four week's duration. *Schmerz* **2015**, *29*, 85–95. [CrossRef]

19. Phillips, M.; Vannabouathong, C.; Devji, T.; Patel, R.; Gomes, Z.; Patel, A.; Dixon, M.; Bhandari, M. Differentiating factors of intra-articular injectables have a meaningful impact on knee osteoarthritis outcomes: A network meta-analysis. *Knee Surg. Sports Traumatol. Arthrosc.* **2020**, *28*, 3031–3039. [CrossRef]
20. Hepper, C.T.; Halvorson, J.J.; Duncan, S.T.; Gregory, A.J.; Dunn, W.R.; Spindler, K.P. The efficacy and duration of intra-articular corticosteroid injection for knee osteoarthritis: A systematic review of level I studies. *J. Am. Acad. Orthop. Surg.* **2009**, *17*, 638–646. [CrossRef]
21. Kijowski, R. Risks and Benefits of Intra-articular Corticosteroid Injection for Treatment of Osteoarthritis: What Radiologists and Patients Need to Know. *Radiology* **2019**, *293*, 664–665. [CrossRef] [PubMed]
22. Sabha, M.; Hochberg, M.C. Non-surgical management of hip and knee osteoarthritis; comparison of ACR/AF and OARSI 2019 and VA/DoD 2020 guidelines. *Osteoarthr. Cartil. Open* **2022**, *4*, 100232. [CrossRef] [PubMed]
23. Cui, Y.; Lin, L.; Wang, Z.; Wang, K.; Xiao, L.; Lin, W.; Zhang, Y. Research trends of platelet-rich plasma therapy on knee osteoarthritis from 2011 to 2021: A review. *Medicine* **2023**, *102*, e32434. [CrossRef] [PubMed]
24. Shen, L.; Yuan, T.; Chen, S.; Xie, X.; Zhang, C. The temporal effect of platelet-rich plasma on pain and physical function in the treatment of knee osteoarthritis: Systematic review and meta-analysis of randomized controlled trials. *J. Orthop. Surg. Res.* **2017**, *12*, 16. [CrossRef]
25. Di Martino, A.; Di Matteo, B.; Papio, T.; Tentoni, F.; Selleri, F.; Cenacchi, A.; Kon, E.; Filardo, G. Platelet-Rich Plasma Versus Hyaluronic Acid Injections for the Treatment of Knee Osteoarthritis: Results at 5 Years of a Double-Blind, Randomized Controlled Trial. *Am. J. Sports Med.* **2019**, *47*, 347–354. [CrossRef]
26. Belk, J.W.; Kraeutler, M.J.; Houck, D.A.; Goodrich, J.A.; Dragoo, J.L.; McCarty, E.C. Platelet-Rich Plasma Versus Hyaluronic Acid for Knee Osteoarthritis: A Systematic Review and Meta-analysis of Randomized Controlled Trials. *Am. J. Sports Med.* **2021**, *49*, 249–260. [CrossRef]
27. Jomphe, C.; Gabriac, M.; Hale, T.M.; Heroux, L.; Trudeau, L.E.; Deblois, D.; Montell, E.; Verges, J.; du Souich, P. Chondroitin sulfate inhibits the nuclear translocation of nuclear factor-kappaB in interleukin-1beta-stimulated chondrocytes. *Basic Clin. Pharmacol. Toxicol.* **2008**, *102*, 59–65. [CrossRef]
28. Aghazadeh-Habashi, A.; Kohan, M.H.; Asghar, W.; Jamali, F. Glucosamine dose/concentration-effect correlation in the rat with adjuvant arthritis. *J. Pharm. Sci.* **2014**, *103*, 760–767. [CrossRef]
29. Li, Y.; Chen, L.; Liu, Y.; Zhang, Y.; Liang, Y.; Mei, Y. Anti-inflammatory effects in a mouse osteoarthritis model of a mixture of glucosamine and chitooligosaccharides produced by bi-enzyme single-step hydrolysis. *Sci. Rep.* **2018**, *8*, 5624. [CrossRef]
30. Waly, N.E.; Refaiy, A.; Aborehab, N.M. IL-10 and TGF-beta: Roles in chondroprotective effects of Glucosamine in experimental Osteoarthritis? *Pathophysiology* **2017**, *24*, 45–49. [CrossRef]
31. Imagawa, K.; de Andres, M.C.; Hashimoto, K.; Pitt, D.; Itoi, E.; Goldring, M.B.; Roach, H.I.; Oreffo, R.O. The epigenetic effect of glucosamine and a nuclear factor-kappa B (NF-kB) inhibitor on primary human chondrocytes—Implications for osteoarthritis. *Biochem. Biophys. Res. Commun.* **2011**, *405*, 362–367. [CrossRef]
32. Wen, Z.H.; Tang, C.C.; Chang, Y.C.; Huang, S.Y.; Hsieh, S.P.; Lee, C.H.; Huang, G.S.; Ng, H.F.; Neoh, C.A.; Hsieh, C.S.; et al. Glucosamine sulfate reduces experimental osteoarthritis and nociception in rats: Association with changes of mitogen-activated protein kinase in chondrocytes. *Osteoarthr. Cartil.* **2010**, *18*, 1192–1202. [CrossRef] [PubMed]
33. Kuptniratsaikul, V.; Dajpratham, P.; Taechaarpornkul, W.; Buntragulpoontawee, M.; Lukkanapichonchut, P.; Chootip, C.; Saengsuwan, J.; Tantayakom, K.; Laongpech, S. Efficacy and safety of Curcuma domestica extracts compared with ibuprofen in patients with knee osteoarthritis: A multicenter study. *Clin. Interv. Aging* **2014**, *9*, 451–458. [CrossRef] [PubMed]
34. Zhu, X.; Sang, L.; Wu, D.; Rong, J.; Jiang, L. Effectiveness and safety of glucosamine and chondroitin for the treatment of osteoarthritis: A meta-analysis of randomized controlled trials. *J. Orthop. Surg. Res.* **2018**, *13*, 170. [CrossRef]
35. Zhu, X.; Wu, D.; Sang, L.; Wang, Y.; Shen, Y.; Zhuang, X.; Chu, M.; Jiang, L. Comparative effectiveness of glucosamine, chondroitin, acetaminophen or celecoxib for the treatment of knee and/or hip osteoarthritis: A network meta-analysis. *Clin. Exp. Rheumatol.* **2018**, *36*, 595–602. [PubMed]
36. Zeng, C.; Wei, J.; Li, H.; Wang, Y.L.; Xie, D.X.; Yang, T.; Gao, S.G.; Li, Y.S.; Luo, W.; Lei, G.H. Effectiveness and safety of Glucosamine, chondroitin, the two in combination, or celecoxib in the treatment of osteoarthritis of the knee. *Sci. Rep.* **2015**, *5*, 16827. [CrossRef] [PubMed]
37. Kwoh, C.K.; Roemer, F.W.; Hannon, M.J.; Moore, C.E.; Jakicic, J.M.; Guermazi, A.; Green, S.M.; Evans, R.W.; Boudreau, R. Effect of oral glucosamine on joint structure in individuals with chronic knee pain: A randomized, placebo-controlled clinical trial. *Arthritis Rheumatol.* **2014**, *66*, 930–939. [CrossRef] [PubMed]
38. Fransen, M.; Agaliotis, M.; Nairn, L.; Votrubec, M.; Bridgett, L.; Su, S.; Jan, S.; March, L.; Edmonds, J.; Norton, R.; et al. Glucosamine and chondroitin for knee osteoarthritis: A double-blind randomised placebo-controlled clinical trial evaluating single and combination regimens. *Ann. Rheum. Dis.* **2015**, *74*, 851–858. [CrossRef] [PubMed]
39. Knapik, J.J.; Pope, R.; Hoedebecke, S.S.; Schram, B.; Orr, R.; Lieberman, H.R. Effects of Oral Glucosamine Sulfate on Osteoarthritis-Related Pain and Joint-Space Changes: Systematic Review and Meta-Analysis. *J. Spec. Oper. Med.* **2018**, *18*, 139–147. [CrossRef]
40. Chiu, H.W.; Li, L.H.; Hsieh, C.Y.; Rao, Y.K.; Chen, F.H.; Chen, A.; Ka, S.M.; Hua, K.F. Glucosamine inhibits IL-1beta expression by preserving mitochondrial integrity and disrupting assembly of the NLRP3 inflammasome. *Sci. Rep.* **2019**, *9*, 5603. [CrossRef]

41. Ohara, H.; Matsumoto, H.; Ito, K.; Iwai, K.; Sato, K. Comparison of quantity and structures of hydroxyproline-containing peptides in human blood after oral ingestion of gelatin hydrolysates from different sources. *J. Agric. Food Chem.* **2007**, *55*, 1532–1535. [CrossRef] [PubMed]
42. Henrotin, Y.; Sanchez, C.; Balligand, M. Pharmaceutical and nutraceutical management of canine osteoarthritis: Present and future perspectives. *Vet. J.* **2005**, *170*, 113–123. [CrossRef] [PubMed]
43. Bagchi, D.; Misner, B.; Bagchi, M.; Kothari, S.C.; Downs, B.W.; Fafard, R.D.; Preuss, H.G. Effects of orally administered undenatured type II collagen against arthritic inflammatory diseases: A mechanistic exploration. *Int. J. Clin. Pharmacol. Res.* **2002**, *22*, 101–110. [PubMed]
44. Tong, T.; Zhao, W.; Wu, Y.Q.; Chang, Y.; Wang, Q.T.; Zhang, L.L.; Wei, W. Chicken type II collagen induced immune balance of main subtype of helper T cells in mesenteric lymph node lymphocytes in rats with collagen-induced arthritis. *Inflamm. Res.* **2010**, *59*, 369–377. [CrossRef]
45. Ohara, H.; Iida, H.; Ito, K.; Takeuchi, Y.; Nomura, Y. Effects of Pro-Hyp, a collagen hydrolysate-derived peptide, on hyaluronic acid synthesis using in vitro cultured synovium cells and oral ingestion of collagen hydrolysates in a guinea pig model of osteoarthritis. *Biosci. Biotechnol. Biochem.* **2010**, *74*, 2096–2099. [CrossRef]
46. Gordon, M.K.; Hahn, R.A. Collagens. *Cell Tissue Res.* **2010**, *339*, 247–257. [CrossRef]
47. Garcia-Coronado, J.M.; Martinez-Olvera, L.; Elizondo-Omana, R.E.; Acosta-Olivo, C.A.; Vilchez-Cavazos, F.; Simental-Mendia, L.E.; Simental-Mendia, M. Effect of collagen supplementation on osteoarthritis symptoms: A meta-analysis of randomized placebo-controlled trials. *Int. Orthop.* **2019**, *43*, 531–538. [CrossRef]
48. Trc, T.; Bohmova, J. Efficacy and tolerance of enzymatic hydrolysed collagen (EHC) vs. glucosamine sulphate (GS) in the treatment of knee osteoarthritis (KOA). *Int. Orthop.* **2011**, *35*, 341–348. [CrossRef]
49. Aitken, D.; Laslett, L.L.; Pan, F.; Haugen, I.K.; Otahal, P.; Bellamy, N.; Bird, P.; Jones, G. A randomised double-blind placebo-controlled crossover trial of HUMira (adalimumab) for erosive hand OsteoaRthritis—The HUMOR trial. *Osteoarthr. Cartil.* **2018**, *26*, 880–887. [CrossRef]
50. Kloppenburg, M.; Ramonda, R.; Bobacz, K.; Kwok, W.Y.; Elewaut, D.; Huizinga, T.W.J.; Kroon, F.P.B.; Punzi, L.; Smolen, J.S.; Vander Cruyssen, B.; et al. Etanercept in patients with inflammatory hand osteoarthritis (EHOA): A multicentre, randomised, double-blind, placebo-controlled trial. *Ann. Rheum. Dis.* **2018**, *77*, 1757–1764. [CrossRef]
51. Ridker, P.M.; Everett, B.M.; Thuren, T.; MacFadyen, J.G.; Chang, W.H.; Ballantyne, C.; Fonseca, F.; Nicolau, J.; Koenig, W.; Anker, S.D.; et al. Antiinflammatory Therapy with Canakinumab for Atherosclerotic Disease. *N. Engl. J. Med.* **2017**, *377*, 1119–1131. [CrossRef] [PubMed]
52. Wang, S.X.; Abramson, S.B.; Attur, M.; Karsdal, M.A.; Preston, R.A.; Lozada, C.J.; Kosloski, M.P.; Hong, F.; Jiang, P.; Saltarelli, M.J.; et al. Safety, tolerability, and pharmacodynamics of an anti-interleukin-1alpha/beta dual variable domain immunoglobulin in patients with osteoarthritis of the knee: A randomized phase 1 study. *Osteoarthr. Cartil.* **2017**, *25*, 1952–1961. [CrossRef] [PubMed]
53. Schnitzer, T.J.; Easton, R.; Pang, S.; Levinson, D.J.; Pixton, G.; Viktrup, L.; Davignon, I.; Brown, M.T.; West, C.R.; Verburg, K.M. Effect of Tanezumab on Joint Pain, Physical Function, and Patient Global Assessment of Osteoarthritis Among Patients With Osteoarthritis of the Hip or Knee: A Randomized Clinical Trial. *JAMA* **2019**, *322*, 37–48. [CrossRef] [PubMed]
54. Berenbaum, F.; Blanco, F.J.; Guermazi, A.; Miki, K.; Yamabe, T.; Viktrup, L.; Junor, R.; Carey, W.; Brown, M.T.; West, C.R.; et al. Subcutaneous tanezumab for osteoarthritis of the hip or knee: Efficacy and safety results from a 24-week randomised phase III study with a 24-week follow-up period. *Ann. Rheum. Dis.* **2020**, *79*, 800–810. [CrossRef] [PubMed]
55. Lane, N.E.; Schnitzer, T.J.; Birbara, C.A.; Mokhtarani, M.; Shelton, D.L.; Smith, M.D.; Brown, M.T. Tanezumab for the treatment of pain from osteoarthritis of the knee. *N. Engl. J. Med.* **2010**, *363*, 1521–1531. [CrossRef]
56. Liu, D.; Kou, X.; Chen, C.; Liu, S.; Liu, Y.; Yu, W.; Yu, T.; Yang, R.; Wang, R.; Zhou, Y.; et al. Circulating apoptotic bodies maintain mesenchymal stem cell homeostasis and ameliorate osteopenia via transferring multiple cellular factors. *Cell Res.* **2018**, *28*, 918–933. [CrossRef] [PubMed]
57. Marks, P.W.; Witten, C.M.; Califf, R.M. Clarifying Stem-Cell Therapy's Benefits and Risks. *N. Engl. J. Med.* **2017**, *376*, 1007–1009. [CrossRef]
58. Jones, I.A.; Togashi, R.; Wilson, M.L.; Heckmann, N.; Vangsness, C.T., Jr. Intra-articular treatment options for knee osteoarthritis. *Nat. Rev. Rheumatol.* **2019**, *15*, 77–90. [CrossRef]
59. Ankrum, J.A.; Ong, J.F.; Karp, J.M. Mesenchymal stem cells: Immune evasive, not immune privileged. *Nat. Biotechnol.* **2014**, *32*, 252–260. [CrossRef]
60. Yubo, M.; Yanyan, L.; Li, L.; Tao, S.; Bo, L.; Lin, C. Clinical efficacy and safety of mesenchymal stem cell transplantation for osteoarthritis treatment: A meta-analysis. *PLoS ONE* **2017**, *12*, e0175449. [CrossRef] [PubMed]
61. Gupta, P.K.; Chullikana, A.; Rengasamy, M.; Shetty, N.; Pandey, V.; Agarwal, V.; Wagh, S.Y.; Vellotare, P.K.; Damodaran, D.; Viswanathan, P.; et al. Efficacy and safety of adult human bone marrow-derived, cultured, pooled, allogeneic mesenchymal stromal cells (Stempeucel(R)): Preclinical and clinical trial in osteoarthritis of the knee joint. *Arthritis Res. Ther.* **2016**, *18*, 301. [CrossRef]
62. Lu, L.; Dai, C.; Du, H.; Li, S.; Ye, P.; Zhang, L.; Wang, X.; Song, Y.; Togashi, R.; Vangsness, C.T.; et al. Intra-articular injections of allogeneic human adipose-derived mesenchymal progenitor cells in patients with symptomatic bilateral knee osteoarthritis: A Phase I pilot study. *Regen. Med.* **2020**, *15*, 1625–1636. [CrossRef] [PubMed]

63. Lamo-Espinosa, J.M.; Mora, G.; Blanco, J.F.; Granero-Molto, F.; Nunez-Cordoba, J.M.; Sanchez-Echenique, C.; Bondia, J.M.; Aquerreta, J.D.; Andreu, E.J.; Ornilla, E.; et al. Intra-articular injection of two different doses of autologous bone marrow mesenchymal stem cells versus hyaluronic acid in the treatment of knee osteoarthritis: Multicenter randomized controlled clinical trial (phase I/II). *J. Transl. Med.* **2016**, *14*, 246. [CrossRef] [PubMed]
64. Bastos, R.; Mathias, M.; Andrade, R.; Bastos, R.; Balduino, A.; Schott, V.; Rodeo, S.; Espregueira-Mendes, J. Intra-articular injections of expanded mesenchymal stem cells with and without addition of platelet-rich plasma are safe and effective for knee osteoarthritis. *Knee Surg. Sports Traumatol. Arthrosc.* **2018**, *26*, 3342–3350. [CrossRef] [PubMed]
65. Delplace, V.; Boutet, M.A.; Le Visage, C.; Maugars, Y.; Guicheux, J.; Vinatier, C. Osteoarthritis: From upcoming treatments to treatments yet to come. *Jt. Bone Spine* **2021**, *88*, 105206. [CrossRef]
66. Cherian, J.J.; Parvizi, J.; Bramlet, D.; Lee, K.H.; Romness, D.W.; Mont, M.A. Preliminary results of a phase II randomized study to determine the efficacy and safety of genetically engineered allogeneic human chondrocytes expressing TGF-beta1 in patients with grade 3 chronic degenerative joint disease of the knee. *Osteoarthr. Cartil.* **2015**, *23*, 2109–2118. [CrossRef]
67. Nixon, A.J.; Grol, M.W.; Lang, H.M.; Ruan, M.Z.C.; Stone, A.; Begum, L.; Chen, Y.; Dawson, B.; Gannon, F.; Plutizki, S.; et al. Disease-Modifying Osteoarthritis Treatment With Interleukin-1 Receptor Antagonist Gene Therapy in Small and Large Animal Models. *Arthritis Rheumatol.* **2018**, *70*, 1757–1768. [CrossRef]
68. Tong, L.; Yu, H.; Huang, X.; Shen, J.; Xiao, G.; Chen, L.; Wang, H.; Xing, L.; Chen, D. Current understanding of osteoarthritis pathogenesis and relevant new approaches. *Bone Res.* **2022**, *10*, 60. [CrossRef]

**Disclaimer/Publisher's Note:** The statements, opinions and data contained in all publications are solely those of the individual author(s) and contributor(s) and not of MDPI and/or the editor(s). MDPI and/or the editor(s) disclaim responsibility for any injury to people or property resulting from any ideas, methods, instructions or products referred to in the content.

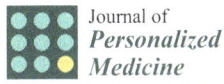

Review

# Current Surgical Techniques in the Treatment of Adult Developmental Dysplasia of the Hip

Anand S. Dhaliwal [1,*], Muzammil Akhtar [1], Daniel I. Razick [1], Arya Afzali [1], Ethan Wilson [1] and Alexander J. Nedopil [1,2,3]

1. College of Medicine, Californa Northstate University, Elk Grove, CA 95757, USA; muzammil.akhtar9106@cnsu.edu (M.A.); daniel.razick10009@cnsu.edu (D.I.R.); arya.afzali7448@cnsu.edu (A.A.); ethan.wilson7202@cnsu.edu (E.W.); ajnedopil@ucdavis.edu (A.J.N.)
2. Orthopädische Klinik König-Ludwig-Haus, Lehrstuhl für Orthopädie der Universität Würzburg, 97074 Würzburg, Germany
3. Department of Biomedical Engineering, University of California, Davis, CA 95616, USA
* Correspondence: anand.Dhaliwal7125@cnsu.edu

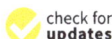

**Abstract:** The surgical protocols currently used for the treatment of developmental dysplasia of the hip (DDH) are varied, with sufficient differences in clinical outcomes that warrant a review of the role of practicing orthopedic surgeons. This paper aims to summarize the current novel techniques within the realm of surgical treatment for adult DDH, thus serving as a guide to surgeons looking to quickly familiarize themselves with available techniques. We performed computer systematic literature searches of the Embase and PubMed databases from 2010 to 2 April 2022. Study parameters as well as their respective patient reported outcomes (PROMs) were described in detail and compiled into diagrams. Two novel techniques were identified for the treatment of borderline or low-grade DDH. Six techniques which included modifications to the Bernese periacetabular osteotomy (PAO) were identified for the treatment of symptomatic DDH. Three techniques which include combinations of arthroscopy and osteotomy were identified for the treatment of DDH with concomitant hip pathologies such as cam deformities. Finally, six techniques, all of which are modifications to total hip arthroplasty (THA), were identified for the treatment of high-grade DDH. The techniques detailed in this review therefore equip surgeons with the necessary knowledge to improve outcomes in patients with varying degrees of DDH.

**Keywords:** hip dysplasia; surgical techniques; osteotomy; total hip arthroplasty; arthroscopy; hip preservation

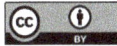

## 1. Introduction

A variety of novel techniques to treat developmental dysplasia of the hip (DDH) in adults have been introduced in the last decade and it is our goal to provide an updated and extensive overview of them for patients with borderline to very severe DDH. Previous systematic reviews examined outcomes of standard techniques to treat adult DDH such as the Bernese periacetabular osteotomy (PAO) or evaluated outcomes for treatment of only borderline adult DDH [1,2]. While these previous studies have provided insightful knowledge regarding the treatment of adult patients with DDH, our aim in this review is to present an extensive overview of each novel technique along with its respective outcomes in treating various degrees of DDH. The novel techniques introduced in this review encompass combinations of arthroscopy, osteotomy, and arthroplasty.

Developmental dysplasia of the hip (DDH) encompasses a multitude of pathologies involving the acetabulum, and occasionally the proximal femur, such as acetabular dysplasia, hip subluxation, true dislocation of the hip, and hip instability. The structural abnormalities present in both the bones and soft tissues surrounding the hip joint can cause the femoral head to move abnormally within the acetabulum which can lead to increased stress on the acetabular rim. In turn, this increases the risk of chondral degeneration and eventually leads to the development of secondary osteoarthritis if left untreated [3,4]. Acetabular dysplasia specifically is defined as inadequate coverage of the femoral head due to a shallow acetabulum and is the subset of DDH pathologies that is more commonly identified in adolescents and adults [5].

Three commonly used methods to determine the severity of DDH in adult patients, which are also used in this review, include the lateral center-edge angle (LCEA) [3], Crowe's method [6] and the Hartofilakidis method [7]. In terms of the anteroposterior (AP) pelvic view, the LCEA is used to assess the coverage of the femoral head by the acetabulum with an LCEA of $25°$–$39°$ being considered normal, that of $20°$–$25°$ being considered borderline, and that of $<20°$ being considered dysplastic [3]. Crowe's method classifies the degree of dysplasia on a scale of I–IV and it states that a larger distance between the medial head–neck junction of the affected hip and the reference line joining both inferior margins of the acetabulum is correlated with a higher degree of dysplasia [6]. Crowe type I–II DDH is generally considered a mild pathology when compared to Crowe III–IV hips which are much more challenging to treat due to extensive distortions to the native anatomy [8,9]. The Hartofilakidis method classifies DDH severity in adults based on the location of the femoral head relative to the acetabulum. Dysplastic hips (type A) have a femoral head that is not dislocated outside of the acetabulum even though subluxation may be present, and these are considered the least severe. Hips with low dislocation (type B) have a partially dislocated femoral head which articulates with a false acetabulum which also covers the true acetabulum to some degree. Hips with high dislocation (type C) have a completely dislocated femoral head which has migrated superoposterioly and has no articulation to the true acetabulum, and this is considered the most severe type [7,10].

THA remains the main treatment for patients with end-stage osteoarthritis secondary to DDH [11]; however, it can be challenging in the setting of DDH due to the anatomy of the dysplastic hip [12]. For this reason, continuous modifications are made to THA in the treatment of DDH to improve results and make it a less demanding procedure. Osteotomy allows early intervention before THA is indicated, and even delays the need for THA by many years [13]. For borderline dysplastic hips (LCEA of $18°$–$25°$) isolated hip arthroscopy is the recommended surgical treatment. However, periacetabular osteotomy (PAO), with or without arthroscopy, may also be beneficial, especially in hips at the upper end of the LCEA spectrum of $18°$–$25°$. Evidence of significant improvements in PROMs is seen in isolated hip arthroscopy, and this is likely due to the effect of addressing intra-articular pathologies, such as labral tears and femoral cam deformities, rather than postoperative radiographic measurements of dysplasia [14,15]. PAO in borderline dysplasia has also shown significant improvements in PROMs; however, categorization of borderline hips with a LCEA of $18°$–$25°$ is overly simplistic as this measurement alone does not take into consideration aspects such as the anterior and posterior head coverage. Additional radiographic measurements such as those of the ACEA, Tönnis acetabular roof angle, the anterior and posterior wall indices, and the femoral epiphyseal acetabular roof (FEAR) index may reveal a much more severe degree of dysplasia than the LCEA criteria suggests [16,17]. Isolated arthroscopy is therefore recommended for patients at the upper end of the LCEA spectrum of $18°$–$25°$ whereas PAO is recommended for hips with more severe dysplasia. PAO is a successful intervention for adult DDH with a 20-year 60% survivorship rate [18]. There have been many modifications made to PAO as well as new osteotomy techniques in recent years. However, many authors have noted intra-articular pathologies causing symptoms after PAO that are not limited to femoroacetabular impingement (FAI) and labral tears which require treatment with additional arthroscopy [19–25].

Treatment options change based on a surgeon's discretion with respect to correcting the specific pathology of a given patient. It is not feasible to compare procedures to identify a universally optimal approach to treatment. Rather, this paper aims to present and summarize the current novel techniques regarding the surgical treatment of adult DDH to quickly familiarize surgeons with available techniques. We hereby present a review of the most common surgical modalities and their respective clinical outcomes pertaining to the treatment of adult DDH.

## 2. Materials and Methods

We followed the guidelines indicated in Preferred Reporting Items for Systematic Reviews and Meta-Analyses (PRISMA). Since we intended to provide an updated review of recent novel techniques for either the femoral and/or acetabular management of adult DDH with PROMs, studies only from 2010 onwards were included. We performed computer systematic literature searches of the Embase and Pubmed databases from 2010 to 2 April 2022. The Embase and Pubmed databases were searched with three different search term criteria. Both databases were first searched with the search terms "hip dysplasia" and "osteotomy" in all fields (title, keywords, abstract, etc.). A second search was conducted with the terms "hip dysplasia" and "arthroscopy" in all fields. A third search was conducted with the terms "hip dysplasia" and "arthroplasty". Searches were performed in two separate databases and very broad search terms were used to ensure we did not miss any articles presenting novel techniques for the treatment of adult DDH. The abstracts were compiled in a reference management software, Endnote.

Two authors independently performed the study selection. Exclusion criteria included systematic reviews, case reports, letters to the editor, conference abstracts, non-English language studies, studies examining salvage/revision procedures, pediatric studies and studies treating hip dysplasia secondary to other diseases (cerebral palsy, Legg–Calve–Perthes disease, septic arthritis, etc.). Duplicates were removed, narrowing down the list of abstracts to 6,630. An Endnote search was performed for the term "technique" in all terms, resulting in 1412 articles. Abstracts of all these articles were screened, and 57 of them discussed a novel surgical technique for the treatment of adult DDH so they were selected for full-text analysis. An additional Endnote search was performed for the keyword "treatment outcome" resulting in 1915 articles. Abstracts of all these articles were screened, and 89 of them discussed outcomes of surgical treatment for adult DDH so they were also selected for full-text analysis. A four-phase flow diagram of the literature selection was prepared according to the guidelines laid down by PRISMA (Figure 1). This diagram depicts the number of studies identified upon the initial search, the number of duplicate studies between both databases, the keywords used to narrow down our search, and reasons for excluding studies after conducting a full-text analysis of the 127 articles.

## 3. Results

### 3.1. Literature Search and Study Characteristics

The total number of references for each database was as follows. The Embase search returned 2979 abstracts; the PubMed search returned 6641 abstracts. Our electronic database search resulted in 9620 publications for review.

A total of 17 articles with level IV evidence were included in the final analysis [26–42]. The sample size ranged from 11–161 patients (12–200 hips). The follow up time ranged from 1 to 18 years. There were six papers introducing modified techniques for THA, of which two techniques included an additional osteotomy. There were nine papers introducing modified PAOs, of which two techniques included an additional arthroscopy. Two papers discussed modified arthroscopy techniques. The additional techniques introduced are the CU (University of Colorado) PAO, the Birmingham interlocking pelvic osteotomy (BIPO), eccentric rotational acetabular osteotomy (ERAO), reverse (anteverting) periacetabular osteotomy (RPAO), Salter osteotomy, capsular arthroplasty, and endoscopic shelf acetabuloplasty.

Most papers reported outcomes using HHS (12 of 17) with three papers reporting the modified Harris Hip Score (mHHS), two papers reporting the Non-Arthritic Hip Score (NAHS), and one paper additionally reporting the UCLA and Tegner scores. Most studies made the diagnosis of hip dysplasia using the Crowe–Ranawat classification (1), Hartofilakidis classification (2), Tonnis classification (3), and the LCEA angle. A diagnosis of Crowe IV or Hartofilakidis type C hips warranted THA interventions.

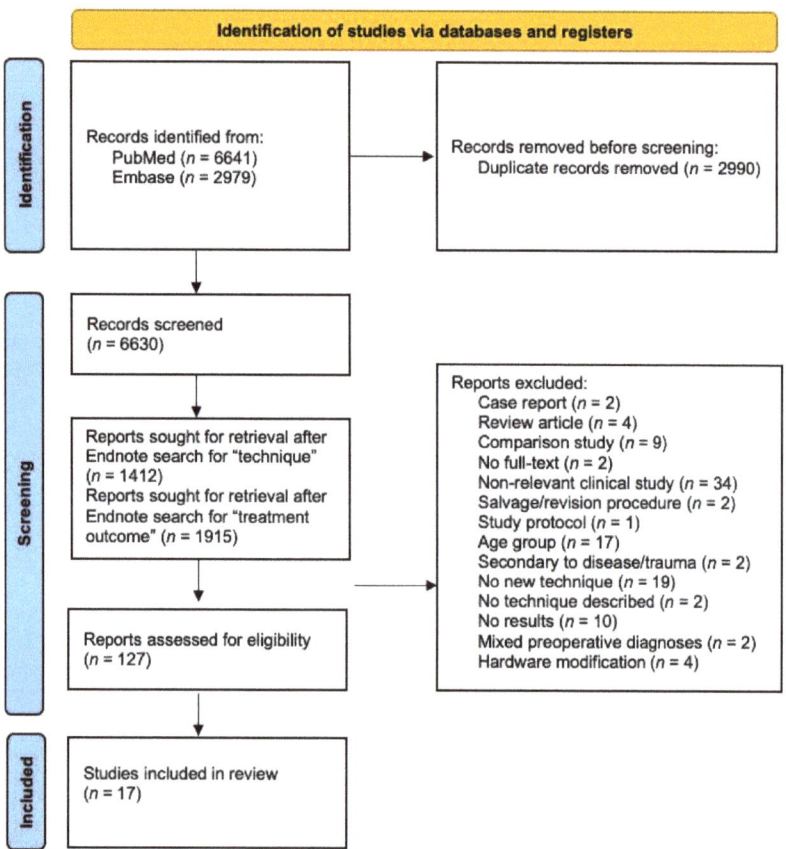

**Figure 1.** Four-phase PRISMA flow diagram.

*3.2. Techniques for Treatment of Borderline or Low-Grade DDH*

While osteotomies and eventually THA are the mainstay treatment for moderate to severe hip dysplasia, low-grade and borderline dysplasia (LCEA between 18°–25°) can be improved via minimally invasive hip arthroscopy as well as a novel technique that incorporates arthroscopy followed by a unique osteotomy [27] (Table 1).

In 2017, Chandrasekaran et al. presented the arthroscopic technique of labral seal restoration with acetabular rim resection and capsular plication for the treatment of borderline hip dysplasia [26]. The authors of this paper present this technique to overcome the iatrogenic micro-instability and macro-instability associated with performing arthroscopy in dysplastic hips [43–45]. Arthroscopy is performed with a standard anterolateral portal, an anterior portal placed under direct visualization, and a distal lateral accessory portal for labral repair. Following diagnostic arthroscopy, concomitant procedures are performed if indicated. In performing capsular plication, the capsule is elevated from the labrum with the use of electrocautery. The preservation of capsular tissue is necessary for later repair. If acetabuloplasty is indicated, very minimal rim resection (2 mm) is performed. To preserve labral tissue, the labrum is not detached from the chondral junction. The labral repair technique (base refixation technique or circumferential suture technique) is chosen based on labral thickness and the quality of tissue. A femoroplasty is performed if a cam deformity is present. The capsule is closed with a suture shuttle technique as described by Chandrasekaran et al. [46]. Capsule closure is completed with four to six sutures via penetration of the acetabular side with a 90-degree SutureLasso while the femoral side of the capsule is penetrated with a sharp bird-beak grasper inferomedially to the acetabular side of the stitch.

Table 1. Study introducing new techniques for treating borderline or low-grade DDH (LCEA between 18°–25°). DDH (developmental dysplasia of the hip); LCEA (lateral-center edge angle); mHHS (modified Harris Hip Score); NAHS (Non Arthritic Hip Score); THA (Total Hip Arthroplasty); LFCN (lateral femoral cutaneous nerve).

| Study | Level of Evidence | Sample | Intervention | Preoperative Diagnosis | Outcome Measures | Results (Mean) | Follow-up (Mean) | Conversion to THA Rate | Complications |
|---|---|---|---|---|---|---|---|---|---|
| Chandra-sekaran, 2017 [26] | IV | 55 hips | Arthroscopy | Borderline DDH (mean LCEA 22.1°) | mHHS | 84.4 (range 80.0 to 88.8) (improvement of 20.7) | 2 years (minimum) | 0% Converted | none |
| Mei-Dan, 2019 [27] | IV | 161 patients (200 hips) | CU (University of Colorado) PAO | DDH (mean LCEA 18.8° ± 6.9) | NAHS | 89.4 (improvement of 33.4) | 2 years | 0% Converted | hardware failures (2) inadvertent intra-articular osteotomy (1) LFCN paresthesia (130 patients) |

A total of 55 procedures were included in this study, of which 11 had a LCEA of between 18°–20°. Arthroscopic findings included labral tear in 55 procedures (100%), chondral defects at the labral–chondral junction in 48 procedures (87.3%), and a LT tear was found in 56.4% of procedures, with complete disruption being evident in 2 patients. There were statistically significant improvements in all PROMs at the 2-year follow-up: improvements in the mHHS, HOSADL, HOS-SSS, and NAHS were 20.7, 17.5, 27.6, and 20.0, respectively. Six patients required revision surgery (two retorn labrums after a traumatic event, two removals of symptomatic loose chondral bodies, and two iliopsoas fractional lengthening for symptomatic internal snapping of the hip), of which three had revisions within two years.

In 2019, Mei-Dan et al. introduced the CU (University of Colorado) PAO, A minimally invasive, two-incision, interlocking periacetabular osteotomy [27]. This novel interlocking PAO developed at the University of Colorado combines the "benefits of the Birmingham interlocking pelvic osteotomy (BIPO) and the Ganz PAO". This technique incorporates the preservation of the posterior column as in the Ganz PAO and the interlocking, two-incision approach of BIPO. A hip arthroscopy is performed on all patients 3–10 days before the PAO. A total of 200 hips from 161 patients were included in this study. The mean follow-up was 20 months (3–33 months). Briefly, 19 hips underwent a concomitant proximal femoral derotational osteotomy. Five revision PAOs were excluded. The mean LCEA improved from 18.8 ± 6.9 preoperatively to 31.5 ± 5.9 at the final follow-up. The mean Tonnis angle improved from 12.0 ± 6.5 preoperatively to 0.6 ± 4.2 at the final follow-up. The mean NAHS improved from 56.0 ± 17.9 preoperatively to 81.2 ± 15.3 at 6 months of follow-up and 87.3 ± 11.9 at 12 months of follow-up. Two hardware failures occurred in the initial development of the technique that required refixation. There was one inadvertent intra-articular osteotomy. Minor complications included lateral femoral cutaneous nerve paresthesia in 130 patients (65%) but this was resolved in 85% of patients in the first 6 months.

*3.3. Techniques for Treatment of Adult DDH (LCEA < 18)*

THA remains the main treatment for patients with end-stage osteoarthritis secondary to DDH [11]. THA can be challenging in the setting of DDH due to the anatomy of the dysplastic hip, including soft tissue retraction, a hypoplastic true acetabulum, a high-riding femur, and a neo acetabulum [12]. For this reason, continuous modifications are made to THA in the treatment of DDH to improve results and make it a less demanding procedure. Osteotomy allows early intervention before THA is indicated, and even delays the need for

THA by many years [13]. The gold standard is PAO, first described by Reihnold Ganz [47]. There have been many modifications made to PAO as well as new osteotomy techniques in recent years. The following table outlines various novel techniques in the treatment of moderate to severe DDH (Table 2).

In 2017, Mei-Dan et al. introduced the Birmingham interlocking pelvic osteotomy for acetabular dysplasia. The authors present a novel triple osteotomy called the Birmingham interlocking pelvic osteotomy (BIPO) [28]. This was originally introduced by Kumar et al. in 1992 in patients with Legg–Calve–Perthes disease [48]. The purpose of developing the BIPO was to improve the safety and reproducibility of pelvic osteotomies and to permit unrestricted postoperative weight bearing with faster recovery. The procedure is broken down into two stages. The first stage is the ischial osteotomy. A posterior mini-incision approach is used. In the second stage, an anterior skin incision is completed as is performed in the Bernese PAO. A total of 116 hips of 100 patients were included in this study. The mean follow-up was 17.5 years. The mean difference from preoperative to postoperative values for the Sourcil angle was 20.6 (18.1–23.0) and the mean difference for LCEA was 30.7 (28.4–33.0). The mean preoperative and postoperative scores were not provided. Only the median scores and mean difference were given. There was a high mean postoperative LCEA score due to intentional overcoverage. In one case, overcoverage caused pathological retroversion which required rim trimming. At the latest follow-up, 38 hips had converted to hip arthroplasty with 34 resurfacing arthroplasties and 4 THAs. Hips not requiring revision had a median OHS of 41 and a median UCLA of 5. Only the first 15 hips had the mean HHS, which improved from a median of 52 preoperatively to a median of 90.5 postoperatively.

Salter osteotomy is a procedure used typically for children between ages 2 and 10 to correct early diagnosed hip dysplasia [49,50]. Schimdutz et al. wanted to assess whether or not Salter osteotomy can correct late-diagnosed hip dysplasia [29]. This surgery was performed as described by Salter in 1978 [51] with a few modifications. Additionally, this is a new technique in the scope of treating adult DDH, making this an important article to include in this review. The following modifications were made:

1. Supine position;
2. Removal of wedge-shaped graft proximal to ASIS;
3. Salter maneuver performed on tilted operating table;
4. Fragment fixation with guide wire;
5. Final acetabular correction in supine position using image intensifier.

A total of 49 hips from 45 patients were included in this study. The mean follow-up was $6.7 \pm 2.7$ years. The mean LCEA improved from $15.5 \pm 9.3$ preoperatively to $35.2 \pm 10$ postoperatively. The mean acetabular index (AI) decreased from $15.4 \pm 6.8$ preoperatively to $4.9 \pm 6.6$ postoperatively. The mean migration percentage improved from $33.2 \pm 9.9\%$ preoperatively to $14.4 \pm 9.3\%$ postoperatively. Two patients had non-union. Four patients had wound impairment due to metal rods. Two patients had deep wound infections. Three patients had nerve injury, one of which was not resolved. At 6.7 years of follow-up, no patients that could be contacted had converted to THA.

**Table 2.** Studies introducing new techniques for treating adult DDH. PAO (periacetabular osteotomy); DVT (deep vein thrombosis); IQR (interquartile range);UCLA (University of California Los Angeles Activity Score).

| Study | Level of Evidence | Sample | Intervention | Preoperative Diagnosis | Outcome Measures | Results (Mean) | Follow-up (Mean) | Conversion to THA Rate | Complications |
|---|---|---|---|---|---|---|---|---|---|
| Mei-Dan, 2017 | IV | 100 patients (116 hips) | BIPO | DDH (median LCEA, 15° +/− 4.5) | HHS | Median: 90.5 (IQR: 90 to 100) (improvement of 38.5) | 17.5 years | 33.04 % Converted | Pulmonary embolism 36 h post-op (1) DVT in opposite limb (2) Non-unions (3) Sciatic nerve palsy (1) LFCN injury (2) Infection (1) Iatrogenic pincer-type femeroacetabular impingement (1) |
| Schmidutz, 2018 | IV | 45 patients (49 hips) | Salter Osteotomy | DDH (mean LCEA, 15.5° ± 9.3°) | HHS | 85.0 ± 11.8 | 6.7 ± 2.7 years | 0% Converted | Non-union (2) Wound impairment due to metal rods (4) Nerve injury (3) |
| Dienst, 2018 | IV | 34 patients (37 hips) | PAO | DDH (mean LCEA, 13.2° ± 7.5) | HHS | 87.6 ± 13.9 | 20.4 ± 10.3 months (median) | 0% Converted | No severe complications Hypoesthesia of peroneal, LFCN, posterior femoral cutaneous, and pudendal nerves (multiple) |
| Khan, 2017 | IV | 151 patients (166 hips) | PAO | DDH (mean LCEA, 14.2° +/− 1.0) | NAHS, UCLA, Tegner scores | 95% CI-NAHS: 58.7 (56.1–63.3) pre-op to 82.9 (80.5–85.3) post-op; UCLA: 4.67 (4.38–4.96) pre-op to 6.83 (6.51–7.16) post-op; Tegner: 2.74 (2.49–2.99) pre-op to 3.78 (3.53–4.03) | 2.8 years | 0.01% Patients Converted | Variable changes in sensation over LFCN distribution Posterior column intra-op crack (1) -stress fractures (12) |
| Shon, 2021 | IV | 49 patients (53 hips) | PAO | DDH (CE angle 2.3 ± 3.3 (0–7)) | HHS | 91.1 (improvement of 29.2) | 11.5 years | 7.0% Converted | Non-union of pubic bone (3) Cross-over signs and ischial spine sign (7) Avulsion fracture of ASIS intra-op (1) |
| Mihalič, 2021 | IV | 35 patients (40 hips) | PAO (electro-magnetic navigation-guided) | DDH (Tönnis grade 0–1) (mean LCEA, 16.35°) | HHS | 88 ± 12 (mean improvement of 38) | 2.87 ± 1.13 years | 0.05% Converted | In control group: peripheral peroneal nerve dysfunction (1) popliteal DVT (1) |

In 2018, Dienst et al. modified the PAO through a double approach [30]. This modification was made based of the authors' experience with Tonnis's triple osteotomy [52]. The goal in this modification is to allow direct vision during the osteotomy of the ischium and the caudal part of the retro acetabular osteotomy. Key modifications are performing the ischial and caudal part of the retroacetabular osteotomy in a "slightly tilted forward" lateral decubitus position and performing the ASIS osteotomy without the exposure of the AIIS, which allows an avoidance of a tenotomy of the rectus femoris tendon. A total of 37 hips in 34 patients were used in this study. The mean follow-up was $20.4 \pm 10.3$ months. The LCEA changed from $13.2 \pm 7.5$ degrees preoperatively to $26.5 \pm 6.7$ degrees. The Tonnis angle reduced from $13.8 \pm 6.5$ degrees to $3.4 \pm 4.4$ degrees. At the final follow-up, the mean HHS was $87.6 \pm 13.9$. A mean preoperative HHS was not provided. There were no major complications. Multiple patients experienced hypothesia of the peroneal nerve, lateral femoral cutaneous nerve, posterior femoral cutaneous nerve, or the pudendal nerve. All cases of hypothesia were resolved over the course of a few weeks up to a maximum of 4 months.

In 2017, Khan et al. introduced a minimally invasive PAO using a modified Smith–Petersen approach [31]. This technique relies upon the usage of specialized osteotomes (Synthes, Salzburg, Austria) and fluoroscopy so as to allow the hip joint capsule to remain unopened. A cohort study was then used to assess compromises in acetabular correction, complication rates, and functional outcomes. In total, 166 hips of 151 patients were included in this study. The mean follow-up was 2.8 years. The mean LCEA improved from 13.4 (13.23–13.57) to 10.1 (9.93–10.27). The mean AI improved from 18.3 (17.2–19.4) to 3.4 (2.59–4.21). There were variable changes in sensation over the distribution of the lateral femoral cutaneous nerve, but these improved drastically over time. One intra-operative crack through the posterior column was noted but did not affect recovery. Stress fractures occurred in 13 hips (7.8%) with 12 fractures in the inferior pubic ramus and one in the posterior column. Conversion to THA occurred in two patients. This was due to the progressive joint space narrowing in one patient as well as pubic non-union and posterior column stress fracture in the other patient. The THA was performed at 2 years and 18 months post-PAO.

Due to the technical difficulties and learning curve associated with the Bernese PAO, many authors [30,53] including Shon et al. [32] have introduced a double approach to PAO. This technique combines the Smith–Petersen and Kocher–Langenbeck approaches. This technique allows a visualization of the posterior column and ischium, whereas the Bernese PAO is performed without direct visualization of these structures. The modified Smith–Petersen technique was used to perform an osteotomy of the pubic bone and ilium, and the Kocher–Langenbeck method was used to perform an osteotomy of the posterior column and ischium. A chest roll positioner was used to rotate the patient between the lateral decubitus position for the posterior incision and the supine position for the anterior incision. A total of 53 hips of 49 patients were included in the study. The average follow-up was 11 years (8–16 years). The average HHS improved from 61.9 before surgery to 91.9 after surgery. Intra-articular osteotomy was observed in two cases due to extension from the osteotomy site. An additional osteotomy was scheduled for one case due to under-correction. Non-union of the pubic bone was observed in three cases. A cross-over sign and ischial spine sign were found in seven cases. An avulsion fracture of the ASIS occurred in one case intra-operatively. No nerve palsies were noted. A 93% survival rate and osteoarthritis progression of 86% was noted at ten years.

In 2021, Mihalič et al. attempted to reintroduce the usage of PAO in Slovenia, originally abandoned in the 1990s due to the steep learning curve and poor midterm outcomes [33]. With many surgeons now taking advantage of intra-operative fluoroscopy to enhance the visualization of the dysplastic hip [47,54]. Mihalič et al. improved on this modification by introducing a electromagnetic navigation (EMN) system and patient-specific templates (PST). The goal was to reduce complications associated with the PAO learning curve and to increase the "accuracy, repeatability, and safety" of the procedure with the following five steps: a CT scan in the DICOM format is uploaded into a medical software application for the creation of a 3D model; the surgeon and a software specialist plan the cuts and acetabular fragment position; the PST is designed to be congruent with the patient's anatomy and with holes for Kirschner wires; the PST is created with biocompatible plastic; finally, the surgery is performed as described by Ganz et al. [47] and soft tissue exposure is determined as described by Siebenrock et al. [53] with modifications for the PST and EMN system.

The EMN system eliminated the time-consuming and unreliable process of using intraoperative fluoroscopy. The authors go on to compare the acetabular fragment placement accuracy between EMN and fluoroscopy (control). A total of 40 hips from 35 patients were included in this study. The mean follow-up was $2.87 \pm 1.13$ years for the EMN group (30 hips) and $6.18 \pm 0.92$ years for the control (fluoroscopy) group (10 hips). Two major complications occurred in the control group (peripheral peroneal nerve dysfunction and popliteal deep vein thrombosis (DVT)) and zero major complications occurred in the EMN group. The only statistically significant difference between the two groups was the average absolute difference in the planned and achieved LCEA and AI, which was $1.2° \pm 1.5°$ and $1.1° \pm 2°$ for the EMN group and $7° \pm 6.1°$ and $6.3° \pm 6.3°$ for the control group ($p = 0.02$; $p = 0.03$). The average HHS value at the final follow-up was $88 \pm 12$ in the EMN group and $86 \pm 14$ in the control group ($p = 0.84$). Direct comparison in a patient that underwent both procedures on opposite hips showed that the difference between the planned and achieved LCEA and AI for the EMN side was $-0.3°$ and $-0.2°$, respectively, while on the control side, the difference between the planned and achieved LCEA and AI was $-8.1°$ and $3.1°$, respectively.

*3.4. Techniques for Treatment of Adult DDH (LCEA < 18) with Concomitant Hip Pathologies*

PAO is a successful intervention for adult DDH with a 20-year 60% survivorship rate [18]. However, many authors have noted intra-articular pathologies causing symptoms after PAO, and the treatment of these pathologies, which includes femoroacetabular impingement and acetabular labral tears, may result in better patient-reported outcomes [34]. PAO with open arthrotomy has been historically favored to treat such pathologies; however, the use of minimally invasive arthroscopy is being explored given the faster recovery time and lower complication rates [36]. The following papers highlight several new modifications to the existing techniques of treating DDH with concomitant intra-articular pathologies (Table 3).

Domb et al.'s early experience with PAO showed a high prevalence of intra-articular abnormalities at the time of PAO [19,25,55]. This led the authors to perform concomitant hip arthroscopies with all PAO procedures at their institution. In this 2015 paper, Domb et al. describe their early experience with this combination of surgical procedures [34]. In this procedure, the arthroscopy is performed prior to the PAO. A traction table is used with the patient supine. Muscle relaxation is also used but stopped during the PAO. A typical arthroscopy is performed with a standard anterolateral portal, a modified anterior portal, and a distal lateral accessory portal. Following diagnostic arthroscopy and treatment, traction is released and the hip is flexed. A femoral osteoplasty is performed using a 5.5 mm round burr. The patient is then transferred to a radiolucent table. The PAO is then performed as modified by Murphy and Millis [55]. A total of 17 patients were included in this study. The mean follow-up was 2.4 years (0.6–3.3 years). Arthroscopic findings included labral repair (12 patients), partial labral debridement (5 patients), iliopsoas fractional lengthening (4 patients), and loose body removal (1 patient). Eight arthroscopic femoral osteoplasty procedures and two open femoral osteoplasty procedures were performed. Three patients underwent microfracture. The mHHS improved from 63.9 preoperatively to 84.1 at the final follow-up ($p < 0.001$); the NAHS improved from 57.7 preoperatively to 79.5 at the final follow-up ($p < 0.001$); the Hip Outcome Score Activities of Daily Living Subscale value improved from 65.4 preoperatively to 80.1 at the final follow-up ($p < 0.005$); and the Hip Outcome Score Sport-Specific Subscale value improved from 37.7 preoperatively to 74.4 at the final follow-up ($p < 0.001$).

Table 3. Studies introducing new techniques for treating adult DDH with concomitant hip pathologies.

| Study | Level of Evidence | Sample | Intervention | Preoperative Diagnosis | Outcome Measures | Results (Mean) | Follow-up (Mean) | Conversion to THA Rate | Complications |
|---|---|---|---|---|---|---|---|---|---|
| Domb, 2015 | IV | 17 patients | PAO+ Arthroscopy | DDH (mean LCEA, 11.15° ± 6.96) | mHHS | 84.1 (improvement of 20.2) | 3 years | 0% Converted | Microfracture (3) Wound infection (2) Pulmonary embolism due to medication noncompliance (1) Partial sciatic nerve palsy (1) Intra-op posterior column fracture (1) |
| Uchida, 2018 | IV | 32 patients (36 hips) | Endoscopic Shelf Acetabuloplasty | DDH (mean LCEA, 16.0° range 5–24) | mHHS | 94.5 ± 8.5 (improvement of 26.1) | 32.3 ± 3 months | 0.02% Converted | Transient LFCN neuropraxia (2) |
| Cho, 2020 | IV | 36 patients (39 hips) | PARO + arthroscopy | DDH (mean LCEA, 8.7° (−9 to 18)) | HHS | 90 (range 68–100) (improvement of 18) | 12.8 ± 1.7 years | 0.03% Converted | Stable, nondisplaced fractures of posterior column intra-op (2) Post-op osteonecrosis of femoral head (1) DVT (1) Heterotrophic ossification (1) Conversion to THA 7.8 years post-op |

The Visual Analog Scale (VAS) score decreased from 5.6 to 2.6 ($p < 0.001$). Two wound infections occurred, one of which was treated pharmacologically while the second required reoperation. Pulmonary embolism occurred in one patient due to noncompliance with the discontinuation of oral contraceptives. One patient suffered from partial sciatic nerve palsy (resolved postoperatively on day 3) and an intra-operative posterior column fracture.

In 2017, Uchida et al. provided the clinical outcomes for their new shelf acetabuloplasty endoscopic technique with arthroscopic chondrolabral and capsular repair with Cam osteoplasty [35] originally described in 2014 [56]. This technique was introduced as an alternative to PAO or RAO for young athletes. While the results for PAO and RAO are satisfactory for moderate to severe dysplasia, the long rehabilitation period and uncertainty regarding return to sports constitutes the need for alternative treatments for this demographic [34,57]. Cam deformities are common in highly active individuals with hip dysplasia [58–60]. Additionally, high stress on a shallow acetabulum can cause labral tears and capsular laxity [60–64]. All these pathologies are addressed with a combination of arthroscopic labral repair, cam osteochondroplasty, capsular plication, and shelf acetabuloplasty in the following sequence: hip arthroscopy as described by Philippon et al. [65], labral repair, traction release and assessment of peripheral compartment for cam lesion, followed by Cam osteochondroplasty using a motorized round burr, capsular plication through the MAP with the hip at 40 degrees of flexion, and finally shelf acetabuloplasty.

Arthroscopic findings included labral tear, ligamentum teres injury and cartilage damage of the femoral head and/or acetabular rim. Two patients reported an increase in UCLA-AS above the preinjury level. A total of 29 of 32 patients returned to sports. The three patients who did not return to sports did not do so due to knee osteoarthritis, shoulder instability, and choice, respectively. The average time for the return to sports was 9 ± 3.5 months. Two patients experienced transient lateral femoral cutaneous nerve neuropraxia. One patient had a fracture of the shelf graft due to returning to sports without physician permission.

In 2020, Cho et al. presented the long-term results of periacetabular rotational osteotomy (PARO) used concomitantly with arthroscopy [36], a technique they originally described in 2011 [66]. The reason for designing this technique was the frequent reports of the disadvantages of arthrotomy in the treatment of intra-articular pathologies of the dysplastic hip [67–70], with expanding indications for the usage of arthroscopy for the dysplastic hip [71]. In this procedure, the osteotomy is performed before the arthroscopy. With the patient in the lateral decubitus position, a curvilinear incision is made 2 cm below the ASIS to 2 cm below the greater trochanter, ending 5 cm below the PSIS. Anterior dissection is performed between the gluteus medius and TFL while a posterior dissection is achieved by splitting the gluteus maximus muscle fibers at the posterior border of the gluteus medius. After the osteotomy of the greater trochanter, arthroscopy is performed while applying manual traction. After addressing any intra-articular pathologies, the surgeon moves on to the PAO. The osteotomy is performed with "specially designed curved osteotomes under image-intensifier control".

A total of 39 hips of 36 patients were included in this study. The mean follow-up was $12.8 \pm 1.7$ years ($153.5 \pm 20.6$; range, 121.8–188.5 months). In total, 39 labral tears were found amongst 39 patients; 15 were degenerative (38.4%), 3 were flap (7.7%), 2 were radial (5.1%), 1 was longitudinal (2.6%), 2 was complex (5.1%), 12 was fibrillar (30.8%), and 4 were intact (10.3%). Various chondral lesions were also identified, including 16 Grade 0 acetabular lesions, 15 Grade 0 femoral lesions, 11 Grade 1 acetabular lesions, 10 Grade 1 femoral lesions, 4 Grade 2 acetabular lesions, 8 Grade 2 femoral lesions, 8 Grade 3 acetabular lesions, and 6 Grade 3 femoral lesions. The average HHS improved from 72 (60–83) preoperatively to 90 (68–100) at the latest follow-up ($p < 0.001$). Complications included two stable, nondisplaced fractures of the posterior column intra-operatively, postoperative osteonecrosis of the femoral head in one hip, one DVT, and one heterotopic ossification around the greater trochanter. Only one hip (2.6%) underwent conversion to THA 7.8 years postoperatively.

### 3.5. Techniques for Treatment of Crowe III–IV or Hartofilakidis Type C Hips

Crowe's method of determining the severity of acetabular dysplasia is the most commonly used one for adult patients. Crowe type I–II DDH is generally considered a mild pathology when compared to Crowe III–IV hips which are much more challenging to treat due to extensive distortions to the native anatomy [8,9]. The Hartofilakidis method is also commonly used to classify DDH severity in adults and is based on the location of the femoral head relative to the acetabulum. Hips with high dislocation (type C) have a completely dislocated femoral head which migrates superoposterioly and has no articulation of the true acetabulum, and this is considered the most severe type [7,10]. In Crowe IV or Hartofilakidis type C hips, THA is often necessary early in life. Challenges include a high hip center, abnormalities in femoral and acetabular anatomy, and soft tissue contractures, and thus require additional osteotomy [72–77]. Benefits include decreased LLD, restoration of the hip center without stretching the sciatic nerve, correcting femoral anteversion, and restoring abductor mechanisms [72,74,76,78,79] (Table 4).

In 2015, Binazzi et al. introduced a new THA technique for treating Crowe IV/Hartofilakidis type C DDH that they have been using and modifying since 1994 [37]. This technique allows the avoidance of the use of subtrochanteric osteotomy by utilizing a two-stage technique of progressively lowering the femur first, and then performing THA. By avoiding osteotomy, patients can potentially gain full limb symmetry and not rely on heel pads or shoe lifts. A total of 11 patients and 12 hips were included in this study. The mean follow-up was 11 years. One patient required revision 5 years after the initial surgery due to infection. The other 11 hips had a mean HHS improvement from $35 \pm 5$ points preoperatively to $85 \pm 5$ points at the final follow-up. For the nine unilateral, unrevised THA patients, leg length discrepancy (LLD) was improved from a mean of $5.7 \pm 1.1$ cm preoperatively to $-0.3 \pm 0.6$ cm postoperatively.

Table 4. Studies introducing new techniques for treating adult Crowe III–IV DDH.

| Study | Level of Evidence | Sample | Intervention | Preoperative Diagnosis | Outcome Measures | Results (Mean) | Follow-up (Mean) | Conversion to THA Rate | Leg Length Discrepancy (Mean) | Leg Length Improvement (Mean) | Complications |
|---|---|---|---|---|---|---|---|---|---|---|---|
| Binazzi, 2015 | IV | 11 patients (12 hips) | THA | Crowe IV/Harto-filakidis type C DDH. HHS: 35±5 | HHS | 85 ± 5 | 11 years | N/A | Pre-Op: 5.7 ± 1.1 cm. Post-Op: −0.3 ± 0.6 cm | −5.4 cm | Revision required 5 years after initial surgery due to infection (1) |
| Montalti, 2018 | IV | 84 hips (80 at final follow-up) | THA | Crowe III–IV DDH; HHS: 35.7 ± 10.4 (range 18.5–46) | HHS | 82.8 ± 9.5 | 15.1 ± 3.1 years | N/A | Crowe III: 19 patients (44%): 0 Longer treated hip: 25 patients (58%), +5 mm (2/12). Shorter treated hip: 4 patients (9%), 4 mm (−2/−8). Crowe IV: 10 patients (27%): 0 Longer treated hip: 12 patients (32%), +3 mm (2/5) Shorter treated hip: 11 patients (30%), −6 mm (−3/−11) | N/A | Traumatic dislocation (1) Sciatic nerve palsy (2) |
| Li, 2018 | IV | 74 patients; 82 hips (49 Crowe III; 33 Crowe IV) | THA | Crowe III–IV DDH; HHS: 42.1 (range 24–71) | HHS | 89.9 (76–100) | 5.1 years | N/A | Average at final follow-up: 0.43 cm (standard deviation, 0.5 cm) | Crowe III: 3.0 cm (1.1–5.5); 2.5 cm (1.1–3.5) Crowe IV: 3.6 cm (1.9–5.5) | Fracture (1) Dislocation (1) Femoral nerve palsy (1) |
| Tahta, 2020 | IV | 77 patients (77 hips) | THA | Crowe III–IV DDH; HHS: 53.9 (49–62) | HHS | 82.7 (76–95) | 38.2 (range 22–52) months | N/A | Pre-op true leg length difference: 4.1 cm (2.9–5.3 cm) | Mean leg lengthening: 3.3 mm (2.4–4.6) | Trendelenburg sign post-op (3) Dislocations (3) Revision due to protrusion development in acetabular cap (1) |
| Kayaalp, 2020 | IV | 41 patients (50 hips) | THA + osteotomy | Crowe III–IV DDH; HHS: 45 ± 14 | HHS | 92 ± 7.8 | 41.6 months | 100% Converted | Pre-op: 2.9 ± 2.5 cm Post-op: 0.8 ± 0.6 cm | −1.9 cm | Trendelenburg sign post-op (2) Non-union which resolved after stem revision due to dislocation after fall (1) |
| Wu, 2020 | IV | 24 patients (26 hips) | THA + osteotomy | Crowe III–IV DDH; HHS: 33.48 ± 9.06 | HHS | 84.61 ± 4.78 | 31.36 ± 10.75 months | 100% Converted | Pre-op: 5.34 ± 1.96 cm Post-op: 1.02 ± 0.77 cm | −4.32 cm | Intraop fractures in 14% of pts Intermuscular vein thrombosis (4) Post-op dislocation due to fall (1) |

In 2018, Montalti et al. developed a THA approach for Crowe III and IV hips that overcomes the issues associated with non-union after femoral osteotomy and with anatomic cup placement in the true acetabulum. This approach is based on a "high center of rotation, a specific implant, and no femoral shortening osteotomy". [38] The aim of this THA is to have a high cup placement without lateralization of the acetabular component. The mean HHS increased from $35.7 \pm 10.4$ preoperatively to $82.8 \pm 9.5$ at the final follow-up. No clinical difference was noted between Crowe III and IV THAs. Survival rate was 90.5%, with five revisions being required. There were three complications noted: one traumatic dislocation and two sciatic nerve palsies.

In 2018, Li et al. introduced a new THA technique for Crowe III and IV hips that allows the avoidance of femoral shortening and relies on direct leverage to the shoulder of the femoral stem for "rapid, safe, and easy" reduction. A total of 82 hips were included in this study [39]. The mean follow-up was 5.1 years. The mean HHS increased from 42.1 (24–71) preoperatively to 89.9 (76–100) at the final follow-up. Preoperative Trendelenburg gait was positive in 42 hips preoperatively, but positive in only two hips at the final follow-up. LLD improved by 3.0 cm (1.1–5.5) and 2.5 cm (1.1–3.5) in Crowe III hips and 3.6 cm (1.9–5.5) in Crowe IV hips. The average LLD at the final follow-up was 0.43 cm (SD 0.5). There were complications in 3 out of 33 hips (fracture, dislocation, and femoral nerve palsy).

In 2020, Kayaalp et al. proposed addressing the issue of instability at the osteotomy site associated with transverse shortening osteotomy by using a Zweymuller rectangular femoral stem [41]. The authors hypothesized that the rectangular femoral stem can be used to overcome the issues of instability due to two reasons: the fit-without-fill principle, "by preserving bone stock and obtaining a biological healing process in highly dysmorphic proximal femurs" and the four-point anchorage to the bone on the axial plane. This will thus prevent the need for a graft or additional osteosynthesis. A total of 50 hips of 41 patients were included in this study. The mean follow-up was 41.6 months. The mean HHS improved from $45 \pm 14$ preoperatively to $92 \pm 7.8$ postoperatively. The mean VAS scores improved from $8.3 \pm 1.7$ preoperatively to $1 \pm 0.9$ postoperatively. The mean LLD improved from $2.9 \pm 2.5$ cm preoperatively to $0.8 \pm 0.6$ postoperatively. The mean stem subsidence was $1.7 \pm 1.2$ mm at six months and $2.1 \pm 1.4$ mm at the final follow-up. A Trendelenburg sign was present in all patients preoperatively but only in two patients postoperatively. Non-union occurred in one patient due to dislocation after a fall. Union occurred after a revision stem in this patient. Intra-operative fractures occurred in 14% of patients.

Wu et al. wanted to address the difficulty of implantation associated with highly dysplastic proximal femurs in DDH [42]. Of the many barriers associated with highly dysplastic femurs, decreased canal size and a thinner cortex are two issues that result in fracture and poor implantation. In 2020, Wu et al. published a modified proximal femoral reconstruction (PFR) technique that allows surgeons to expand the canal volume seamlessly and reduce the femur length at the surgeon's discretion. This technique provides comparable results to those of subtrochanteric transverse osteotomy. A total of 26 hips from 24 patients with Crowe III–IV DDH were included in this study. Follow-up was at 3 and 12 months. The mean HHS improved from $33.48 \pm 9.06$ preoperatively to $84.61 \pm 4.78$ immediately postoperation and $90.84 \pm 4.96$ at 3 months. The VAS score was $6.92 \pm 0.93$ preoperatively, which changed to $1.19 \pm 0.80$ at 12 months of follow-up. Lower limb discrepancy decreased from $5.34 \pm 1.96$ cm preoperatively to $1.02 \pm 0.77$ cm postoperatively. At the last follow-up, there were no cases of non-union or prosthesis loosening. The average union time was $4.35 \pm 1.24$ months. Complications included four patients developing intermuscular vein thrombosis and one patient having a dislocation at 1 month postoperation due to a fall.

## 4. Discussion

Depending on severity of dysplasia and the presence of intra-articular pathologies, choosing the optimal surgical approach can be a challenge. Factors such as recovery times, complications and PROMs should be considered. This paper comprehensively and concisely summarizes several novel techniques used in the treatment of DDH and outlines the pertinent considerations that a surgeon should evaluate before a surgical intervention is performed. This review can be consulted to efficiently choose between current techniques in treating DDH.

For patients with borderline hip dysplasia, defined in this case as a LCEA between 18°–25°, two novel techniques for treatment were identified: arthroscopy and the CU PAO. Chandrasekaran et al. [26]. presented a novel method of performing arthroscopic labral seal restoration with minimal acetabular rim resection and capsular plication to overcome iatrogenic the micro-instability and macro-instability commonly associated with performing arthroscopy in dysplastic hips. Importantly, there were no associated complications and no conversions to THA at a minimum of two years of follow-up; however, 6/55 hips required revision surgery. Surgeons should therefore be aware of the potential need for revision surgery when performing arthroscopy on borderline dysplastic hips. The authors of this study recommend this technique for patients in which PAO is too invasive and because of evidence that traditional hip arthroscopy has the potential to exacerbate the instability of the hip [1,15,43,44]. Mei-Dan et al. [27] introduced the CU PAO, a novel technique for borderline dysplastic hips in which routine hip arthroscopy is performed 3–10 days prior to the modified PAO. The authors recommend this technique for patients with substantial hip instability in whom isolated arthroscopy has a high risk of failure. At a two-year follow-up, the CU PAO showed no conversions to THA; however, complications included hardware failure in two patients during the initial development of the technique and an inadvertent intra-articular osteotomy in another patient. Despite three complications, there were significant improvements in the NAHS postoperation.

For less dysplastic hips (Crowe I–III/Hartofilakidis type A–B) and hips that had not progressed to severe osteoarthritis, modified acetabular osteotomies were performed, with the majority of these studies addressing either improving visualization or creating minimally invasive approaches to PAOs. Mei-Dan et al. [28]. created their BIPO, a triple osteotomy, to improve safety, reproducibility, and permit unrestricted postoperative weight bearing. Despite an excellent median HHS of 90.5 at the latest follow-up, 33% of hips converted to THA; however, this may be attributed to the long follow-up of 17.5 years in which case the conversion rate is similar to that of the standard Bernese PAO [80]. Additionally, the Salter osteotomy was introduced into the adult population by Schimdutz et al. [29]; however, due to its limited range of acetabular correction, the Bernese PAO was deemed preferable. Dienst et al. [30] and Shon et al. [32] both introduced modified PAOs to allow better visualization when performing osteotomies. The mean HHS values at the latest follow-up were 87.6 and 91.9, respectively, with major complications of pubic bone nonunion [3] and an avulsion fracture of the ASIS [1] occurring in the study by Shon et al. Khan et al. [31] presented a minimally invasive approach to PAO which left the hip joint capsule unopened. Stress fracture was the most common complication [13], with 12 occurring in the inferior pubic ramus. Mihalic et al. [33] built upon intra-operative fluoroscopy by introducing the EMN system and PST which successfully reduced complications associated with the steep learning curve of the Bernese PAO.

In addition to hip dysplasia, in patients with concomitant intra-articular pathologies, such as labral tears and cam deformities, modified combinations of PAO and arthroscopy were identified in this review. Domb et al. [34] described a similar level of complications with improved outcomes in patients undergoing arthroscopy to treat intra-articular pathologies followed by PAO compared to those undergoing isolated PAO. Similarly, Cho et al. [36] described a combined arthroscopy with PARO, allowing the treatment of labral tears and chondral lesions, followed by the osteotomy. Between these two studies, there was only one conversion to THA at 7.8 years in the study by Cho et al., along with excellent improvements in PROs in both studies. Uchida et al. [35] introduced a novel technique combining arthroscopic labral repair, cam osteochondroplasty, capsular plication, and shelf acetabuloplasty. This technique is especially beneficial for athletes for whom PAO alone is not sufficient due to the likely presence of cam deformities, labral tears, and capsular laxity. All athletes in this cohort returned to sports rather quickly at an average of 9 ± 3.5 months, with only three not returning due to non-hip-related reasons. Though a paucity of literature exists that examines the outcome of combined PAO and arthroscopy, these three studies highlight their success, especially in patients with concomitant intra-articular pathologies. Even at a long-term follow-up of nearly 13 years by Cho et al., hip survivorship, defined as not converting to THA, was 97.4%.

For patients with severe dysplasia (Crowe III–IV/Hartofilakidis type C), variations of THA remain the gold standard, while THA with osteotomy has been recently explored as well. Binazzi et al. [37] modified the standard THA by utilizing a two-stage technique prior to THA and avoiding osteotomy. Only one patient underwent revision due to infection. Montalti et al. [38] created a modification to allow high cup placement without acetabular component lateralization. Despite a survival rate of 90.5%, five revisions were required with three severe complications noted. Li et al. [39] modified THA by aiming to avoid femoral shortening, resulting in improved leg length discrepancy along with only three complications. Kayaalp et al. [41] modified THA with a novel osteotomy approach in order to address osteotomy site instability, preventing the need for graft or additional osteosynthesis. The mean HHS improved significantly though intra-operative fractures were noted in 14% of patients. An additional THA plus osteotomy modification was introduced by Wu et al. [42] to address the implantation difficulty associated with highly dysplastic proximal femurs using a proximal femoral reconstruction technique. At the latest follow-up, no cases of non-union or prosthesis loosening were noted, though complications included intermuscular vein thrombosis in four patients and dislocation secondary to a fall in one patient. In all studies, postoperative HHS was categorized as good or excellent as the mean scores ranged from 82.8–92 [80]. To provide a relative comparison, patients undergoing traditional THA report similar postoperative HHS, with mean scores ranging from 75–95.6 [81]. Additionally, complications in these studies were similar to those seen in standard THAs such as wound infections, thromboembolic disease, nerve injury, periprosthetic fracture, and dislocation or recurrent instability [82]. Overall complication rates were, however, lower in these studies with a range of 3.6–21.9% compared to those of standard THA [83].

## 5. Conclusions

The surgical protocols currently used for the treatment of DDH are varied, with sufficient differences in clinical outcomes that warrant a review on the part of all practicing orthopedic surgeons. Rapid familiarization must accompany the advent of new and novel techniques, effectively broadening providers' knowledge and skill sets with respect to treating DDH. While studies evaluating specific treatment outcomes with regard to current techniques and investigations into the pathogenesis of DDH are numerous, reviews that provide surgeons with an overview of clinical outcomes for different techniques are necessary to maintaining or even elevating the current standard of care. Discrepancies in patient outcomes can be better understood and mitigated with reviews such as this that recapitulate the significant findings of more targeted studies in a comprehensive manner.

The novel techniques presented in this review are categorized by the severity of adult DDH along with presence of concomitant pathologies. Two novel techniques, modified arthroscopy and PAO, were identified for the treatment of borderline or low-grade DDH. Six techniques, most of which were modifications to the Bernese PAO, were identified for the treatment of standard symptomatic DDH. Three techniques which include combinations of arthroscopy and osteotomy were identified for the treatment of DDH with concomitant hip pathologies such as cam deformities. Six techniques, all of which were modifications to THA, were identified for treatment of severe high-grade DDH. The authors of each technique have also made attempts to improve on the various complications and difficulties associated with surgically treating a dysplastic hip. For surgeons looking to adopt new techniques, it is important to identify areas of improvement that can be addressed by these novel methods, as they vary from paper to paper.

## 6. Limitations

This paper has its limitations. While a thorough search was performed with three separate search terms on two separate databases, there is the possibility that some novel techniques were skipped over in the search process. Additionally, the authors of this paper only included articles that included patient follow-ups. There are novel surgical techniques in the literature that do not have patient-reported outcomes available at the moment. Such papers were excluded from the literature search. This paper also does not include a real systematic comparison of the techniques, as the variability of procedures and demographics do not allow us to make direct comparisons. Ultimately, it is difficult to highlight which one of these procedures is superior to the others. Rather, we hope that the information provided allows surgeons to investigate procedures that will assist in improving outcomes in their own patient subsets.

**Author Contributions:** Conceptualization, A.S.D.; methodology, A.S.D. and A.J.N.; software, A.S.D.; validation, A.J.N. and A.S.D.; formal analysis, A.S.D., M.A., D.I.R. and A.A.; investigation, A.J.N., A.S.D., A.A. and EW.; data curation, A.S.D. and A.A.; writing—original draft preparation, A.S.D., M.A., D.I.R., A.A. and E.W.; writing—review and editing, A.J.N., M.A., D.I.R., A.S.D., A.A. and E.W.; visualization, A.J.N. and A.S.D.; supervision, A.J.N. All authors have read and agreed to the published version of the manuscript.

**Funding:** This research received no external funding.

**Institutional Review Board Statement:** Not applicable.

**Informed Consent Statement:** Not applicable.

**Data Availability Statement:** Not applicable.

**Conflicts of Interest:** The authors declare no conflict of interest.

## References

1. Lodhia, P.; Chandrasekaran, S.; Gui, C.; Darwish, N.; Suarez-Ahedo, C.; Domb, B.G. Open and Arthroscopic Treatment of Adult Hip Dysplasia: A Systematic Review. *Arthroscopy* **2016**, *32*, 374–383. [CrossRef] [PubMed]
2. Kraeutler, M.J.; Safran, M.R.; Scillia, A.J.; Ayeni, O.R.; Garabekyan, T.; Mei-Dan, O. A Contemporary Look at the Evaluation and Treatment of Adult Borderline and Frank Hip Dysplasia. *Am. J. Sport. Med.* **2020**, *48*, 2314–2323. [CrossRef] [PubMed]
3. Schmitz, M.R.; Murtha, A.S.; Clohisy, J.C. ANCHOR Study Group. Developmental Dysplasia of the Hip in Adolescents and Young Adults. *J. Am. Acad. Orthop. Surg.* **2020**, *28*, 91–101. [CrossRef]
4. Vaquero-Picado, A.; González-Morán, G.; Garay, E.G.; Moraleda, L. Developmental dysplasia of the hip: Update of management. *EFORT Open Rev.* **2019**, *4*, 548–556. [CrossRef] [PubMed]
5. Yang, S.; Zusman, N.; Lieberman, E.; Goldstein, R.Y. Developmental Dysplasia of the Hip. *Pediatrics* **2019**, *143*, e20181147. [CrossRef]
6. Crowe, J.F.; Mani, V.J.; Ranawat, C.S. Total hip replacement in congenital dislocation and dysplasia of the hip. *J. Bone Joint Surg. Am.* **1979**, *61*, 15–23. [CrossRef]
7. Hartofilakidis, G.; Stamos, K.; Ioannidis, T.T. Low friction arthroplasty for old untreated congenital dislocation of the hip. *J. Bone Joint Surg. Br.* **1988**, *70*, 182–186. [CrossRef]
8. Liu, Z.Y.; Zhang, J.; Wu, S.T.; Li, Z.Q.; Xu, Z.H.; Zhang, X.; Zhou, Y.; Zhang, Y. Direct Anterior Approach in Crowe Type III-IV Developmental Dysplasia of the Hip: Surgical Technique and 2 years Follow-up from Southwest China. *Orthop. Surg.* **2020**, *12*, 1140–1152. [CrossRef]
9. Chen, M.; Gittings, D.J.; Yang, S.; Liu, X. Total Hip Arthroplasty for Crowe Type IV Developmental Dysplasia of the Hip Using a Titanium Mesh Cup and Subtrochanteric Femoral Osteotomy. *Iowa Orthop. J.* **2018**, *38*, 191–195.
10. Jawad, M.U.; Scully, S.P. In brief: Crowe's classification: Arthroplasty in developmental dysplasia of the hip. *Clin. Orthop. Relat. Res.* **2011**, *469*, 306–308. [CrossRef]
11. Sanchez-Sotelo, J.; Berry, D.J.; Trousdale, R.T.; Cabanela, M.E. Surgical treatment of developmental dysplasia of the hip in adults: II. Arthroplasty options. *J. Am. Acad. Orthop. Surg.* **2002**, *10*, 334–344. [CrossRef] [PubMed]
12. Argenson, J.N.; Flecher, X.; Parratte, S.; Aubaniac, J.M. Anatomy of the dysplastic hip and consequences for total hip arthroplasty. *Clin. Orthop. Relat. Res.* **2007**, *465*, 40–45. [CrossRef] [PubMed]
13. Sohatee, M.A.; Ali, M.; Khanduja, V.; Malviya, A. Does hip preservation surgery prevent arthroplasty? Quantifying the rate of conversion to arthroplasty following hip preservation surgery. *J. Hip Preserv. Surg.* **2020**, *7*, 168–182. [CrossRef] [PubMed]
14. Wyatt, M.C.; Beck, M. The management of the painful borderline dysplastic hip. *J. Hip Preserv. Surg.* **2018**, *5*, 105–112. [CrossRef]
15. Byrd, J.W.; Jones, K.S. Hip arthroscopy in the presence of dysplasia. *Arthroscopy* **2003**, *19*, 1055–1060. [CrossRef]

16. McClincy, M.P.; Wylie, J.D.; Kim, Y.J.; Millis, M.B.; Novais, E.N. Periacetabular Osteotomy Improves Pain and Function in Patients with Lateral Center-edge Angle Between 18° and 25°, but Are These Hips Really Borderline Dysplastic? *Clin. Orthop. Relat. Res.* **2019**, *477*, 1145–1153. [CrossRef]
17. Nepple, J.J.; Fowler, L.M.; Larson, C.M. Decision-making in the Borderline Hip. *Sport. Med. Arthrosc. Rev.* **2021**, *29*, 15–21. [CrossRef]
18. Steppacher, S.D.; Tannast, M.; Ganz, R.; Siebenrock, K.A. Mean 20-year followup of Bernese periacetabular osteotomy. *Clin. Orthop. Relat. Res.* **2008**, *466*, 1633–1644. [CrossRef]
19. Redmond, J.M.; Gupta, A.; Stake, C.E.; Domb, B.G. The prevalence of hip labral and chondral lesions identified by method of detection during periacetabular osteotomy: Arthroscopy versus arthrotomy. *Arthroscopy* **2014**, *30*, 382–388. [CrossRef]
20. Matta, J.M.; Stover, M.D.; Siebenrock, K. Periacetabular osteotomy through the Smith-Petersen approach. *Clin. Orthop. Relat. Res.* **1999**, *363*, 21–32.
21. Ginnetti, J.G.; Pelt, C.E.; Erickson, J.A.; Van Dine, C.; Peters, C.L. Prevalence and treatment of intraarticular pathology recognized at the time of periacetabular osteotomy for the dysplastic hip. *Clin. Orthop. Relat. Res.* **2013**, *471*, 498–503. [CrossRef] [PubMed]
22. Siebenrock, K.A.; Schoeniger, R.; Ganz, R. Anterior femoroacetabular impingement due to acetabular retroversion. Treatment with periacetabular osteotomy. *J. Bone Joint Surg. Am.* **2003**, *85*, 278–286. [CrossRef] [PubMed]
23. Fujii, M.; Nakashima, Y.; Yamamoto, T.; Mawatari, T.; Motomura, G.; Iwamoto, Y.; Noguchi, Y. Effect of intraarticular lesions on the outcome of periacetabular osteotomy in patients with symptomatic hip dysplasia. *J. Bone Joint Surg. Br.* **2011**, *93*, 1449–1456. [CrossRef] [PubMed]
24. Albers, C.E.; Steppacher, S.D.; Ganz, R.; Tannast, M.; Siebenrock, K.A. Impingement adversely affects 10-year survivorship after periacetabular osteotomy for DDH. *Clin. Orthop. Relat. Res.* **2013**, *471*, 1602–1614. [CrossRef]
25. Domb, B.G.; Lareau, J.M.; Baydoun, H.; Botser, I.; Millis, M.B.; Yen, Y.M. Is intraarticular pathology common in patients with hip dysplasia undergoing periacetabular osteotomy? *Clin. Orthop. Relat. Res.* **2014**, *472*, 674–680. [CrossRef]
26. Chandrasekaran, S.; Darwish, N.; Martin, T.J.; Suarez-Ahedo, C.; Lodhia, P.; Domb, B.G. Arthroscopic Capsular Plication and Labral Seal Restoration in Borderline Hip Dysplasia: 2-Year Clinical Outcomes in 55 Cases. *Arthroscopy* **2017**, *33*, 1332–1340. [CrossRef]
27. Mei-Dan, O.; Welton, K.L.; Kraeutler, M.J.; Young, D.A.; Raju, S.; Garabekyan, T. The CU PAO: A Minimally Invasive, 2-Incision, Interlocking Periacetabular Osteotomy: Technique and Early Results. *J. Bone Joint Surg. Am.* **2019**, *101*, 1495–1504. [CrossRef]
28. Mei-Dan, O.; Jewell, D.; Garabekyan, T.; Brockwell, J.; Young, D.A.; McBryde, C.W.; O'Hara, J.N. The Birmingham Interlocking Pelvic Osteotomy for acetabular dysplasia: 13-to 21-year survival outcomes. *Bone Joint J.* **2017**, *99*, 724–731. [CrossRef]
29. Schmidutz, F.; Roesner, J.; Niethammer, T.R.; Paulus, A.C.; Heimkes, B.; Weber, P. Can Salter osteotomy correct late diagnosed hip dysplasia: A retrospective evaluation of 49 hips after 6.7 years? *Orthop. Traumatol. Surg. Res.* **2018**, *104*, 637–643. [CrossRef]
30. Dienst, M.; Goebel, L.; Birk, S.; Kohn, D. Bernese periacetabular osteotomy through a double approach: Simplification of a surgical technique. *Oper. Orthop. Traumatol.* **2018**, *30*, 342–358. [CrossRef]
31. Khan, O.H.; Malviya, A.; Subramanian, P.; Agolley, D.; Witt, J.D. Minimally invasive periacetabular osteotomy using a modified Smith-Petersen approach: Technique and early outcomes. *Bone Joint J.* **2017**, *99*, 22–28, Erratum in *Bone Joint J.* **2017**, *99*, 702–704. [CrossRef] [PubMed]
32. Shon, H.C.; Park, W.S.; Chang, J.S.; Byun, S.E.; Son, D.W.; Park, H.J.; Ha, S.H.; Park, K.T.; Park, J.H. Long-term results of Bernese periacetabular osteotomy using a dual approach in hip dysplasia. *Arch. Orthop. Trauma Surg.* **2023**, *143*, 591–602. [CrossRef] [PubMed]
33. Mihalič, R.; Brumat, P.; Trebše, R. Bernese peri-acetabular osteotomy performed with navigation and patient-specific templates is a reproducible and safe procedure. *Int. Orthop.* **2021**, *45*, 883–889. [CrossRef] [PubMed]
34. Domb, B.G.; LaReau, J.M.; Hammarstedt, J.E.; Gupta, A.; Stake, C.E.; Redmond, J.M. Concomitant Hip Arthroscopy and Periacetabular Osteotomy. *Arthroscopy* **2015**, *31*, 2199–2206. [CrossRef] [PubMed]
35. Uchida, S.; Hatakeyama, A.; Kanezaki, S.; Utsunomiya, H.; Suzuki, H.; Mori, T.; Chang, A.; Matsuda, D.K.; Sakai, A. Endoscopic shelf acetabuloplasty can improve clinical outcomes and achieve return to sports-related activity in active patients with hip dysplasia. *Knee Surg. Sport. Traumatol. Arthrosc.* **2018**, *26*, 3165–3177. [CrossRef]
36. Cho, Y.J.; Kim, K.I.; Kwak, S.J.; Ramteke, A.; Yoo, M.C. Long-Term Results of Periacetabular Rotational Osteotomy Concomitantly with Arthroscopy in Adult Acetabular Dysplasia. *J. Arthroplast.* **2020**, *35*, 2807–2812. [CrossRef]
37. Binazzi, R. Two-Stage Progressive Femoral Lowering Followed by Cementless Total Hip Arthroplasty for Treating Crowe IV-Hartofilakidis Type 3 Developmental Dysplasia of the Hip. *J. Arthroplast.* **2015**, *30*, 790–796. [CrossRef]
38. Montalti, M.; Castagnini, F.; Giardina, F.; Tassinari, E.; Biondi, F.; Toni, A. Cementless Total Hip Arthroplasty in Crowe III and IV Dysplasia: High Hip Center and Modular Necks. *J. Arthroplast.* **2018**, *33*, 1813–1819. [CrossRef]
39. Li, H.; Yuan, Y.; Xu, J.; Chang, Y.; Dai, K.; Zhu, Z. Direct Leverage for Reducing the Femoral Head in Total Hip Arthroplasty Without Femoral Shortening Osteotomy for Crowe Type 3 to 4 Dysplasia of the Hip. *J. Arthroplast.* **2018**, *33*, 794–799. [CrossRef]
40. Tahta, M.; Isik, C.; Uluyardimci, E.; Cepni, S.; Oltulu, I. Total hip arthroplasty without subtrochanteric femoral osteotomy is possible in patients with Crowe III/IV developmental dysplasia: Total hip arthroplasty without femoral osteotomy. *Arch. Orthop. Trauma Surg.* **2020**, *140*, 409–413. [CrossRef]

41. Kayaalp, M.E.; Can, A.; Erdogan, F.; Ozsahin, M.K.; Aydingoz, O.; Kaynak, G. Clinical and Radiological Results of Crowe Type 3 or 4 Dysplasia Patients Operated on With Total Hip Arthroplasty Using a Cementless Rectangular Femoral Component Without Fixating or Grafting the Transverse Osteotomy Site. *J. Arthroplast.* **2020**, *35*, 2537–2542. [CrossRef] [PubMed]
42. Wu, K.; Zhang, X.; Chen, M.; Shang, X. Restoration of Proximal Femoral Anatomy during Total Hip Arthroplasty for High Developmental Dysplasia of the Hip: An Original Technique. *Orthop. Surg.* **2020**, *12*, 343–350. [CrossRef] [PubMed]
43. Austin, D.C.; Horneff, J.G., 3rd; Kelly, J.D., 4th. Anterior hip dislocation 5 months after hip arthroscopy. *Arthroscopy* **2014**, *30*, 1380–1382. [CrossRef]
44. Ross, J.R.; Clohisy, J.C.; Baca, G.; Sink, E. ANCHOR Investigators. Patient and disease characteristics associated with hip arthroscopy failure in acetabular dysplasia. *J. Arthroplast.* **2014**, *29* (Suppl. S9), 160–163. [CrossRef]
45. Parvizi, J.; Bican, O.; Bender, B.; Mortazavi, S.J.; Purtill, J.J.; Erickson, J.; Peters, C. Arthroscopy for labral tears in patients with developmental dysplasia of the hip: A cautionary note. *J. Arthroplast.* **2009**, *24* (Suppl. S6), 110–113. [CrossRef]
46. Chandrasekaran, S.; Vemula, S.P.; Martin, T.J.; SuarezAhedo, C.; Lodhia, P.; Domb, B.G. Arthroscopic technique of capsular pli-cation for the treatment of hip instability. *Arthrosc. Tech.* **2015**, *4*, e163–e167. [CrossRef] [PubMed]
47. Ganz, R.; Klaue, K.; Vinh, T.S.; Mast, J.W. A new periacetabular osteotomy for the treatment of hip dysplasias. Technique and preliminary results. *Clin. Orthop. Relat. Res.* **1988**, *232*, 26–36. [CrossRef]
48. Kumar, D.; Bache, C.E.; O'Hara, J.N. Interlocking triple pelvic osteotomy in severe Legg-Calvé-Perthes disease. *J. Pediatr. Orthop.* **2002**, *22*, 464–470. [CrossRef] [PubMed]
49. Ning, B.; Yuan, Y.; Yao, J.; Zhang, S.; Sun, J. Analyses of outcomes of one-stage operation for treatment of late-diagnosed developmental dislocation of the hip: 864 hips followed for 3.2 to 8.9 years. *BMC Musculoskelet. Disord.* **2014**, *15*, 401. [CrossRef] [PubMed]
50. Arslan, H.; Sucu, E.; Ozkul, E.; Gem, M.; Kisin, B. Should routine pelvic osteotomy be added to the treatment of DDH after 18 months? *Acta Orthop. Belg.* **2014**, *80*, 205–210.
51. Salter, R.B. The classic. Innominate osteotomy in the treatment of congenital dislocation and subluxation of the hip. *Clin. Orthop. Relat. Res.* **1978**, *137*, 2–14.
52. Zahedi, A.R.; Lüring, C.; Janßen, D. Die 3-fache Beckenosteotomie nach Tönnis u. Kalchschmidt [Tönnis and Kalchschmidt triple pelvic osteotomy]. *Orthopade* **2016**, *45*, 673–677. [CrossRef] [PubMed]
53. Siebenrock, K.A.; Steppacher, S.D.; Tannast, M.; Büchler, L. Anteverting Periacetabular Osteotomy for Acetabular Retroversion. *JBJS Essent. Surg. Tech.* **2015**, *5*, e1. [CrossRef] [PubMed]
54. Clohisy, J.C.; Schutz, A.L.; St John, L.; Schoenecker, P.L.; Wright, R.W. Periacetabular osteotomy: A systematic literature review. *Clin. Orthop. Relat. Res.* **2009**, *467*, 2041–2052. [CrossRef]
55. Murphy, S.B.; Millis, M.B. Periacetabular osteotomy without abductor dissection using direct anterior exposure. *Clin. Orthop. Relat. Res.* **1999**, *364*, 92–98. [CrossRef]
56. Uchida, S.; Wada, T.; Sakoda, S.; Ariumi, A.; Sakai, A.; Iida, H.; Nakamura, T. Endoscopic shelf acetabuloplasty combined with labral repair, cam osteochondroplasty, and capsular plication for treating developmental hip dysplasia. *Arthrosc. Tech.* **2014**, *3*, e185–e191. [CrossRef]
57. Ettinger, M.; Berger, S.; Floerkemeier, T.; Windhagen, H.; Ezechieli, M. Sports activity after treatment of residual hip dysplasia with triple pelvic osteotomy using the Tönnis and Kalchschmidt technique. *Am. J. Sport. Med.* **2015**, *43*, 715–720. [CrossRef]
58. Siebenrock, K.A.; Ferner, F.; Noble, P.C.; Santore, R.F.; Werlen, S.; Mamisch, T.C. The cam-type deformity of the proximal femur arises in childhood in response to vigorous sporting activity. *Clin. Orthop. Relat. Res.* **2011**, *469*, 3229–3240. [CrossRef]
59. Paliobeis, C.P.; Villar, R.N. The prevalence of dysplasia in femoroacetabular impingement. *Hip Int.* **2011**, *21*, 141–145. [CrossRef]
60. Yamamuro, T.; Ishida, K. Recent advances in the prevention, early diagnosis, and treatment of congenital dislocation of the hip in Japan. *Clin. Orthop. Relat. Res.* **1984**, *184*, 34–40. [CrossRef]
61. Fujii, M.; Nakashima, Y.; Jingushi, S. Intraarticular findings in symptomatic developmental dysplasia of the hip. *J. Pediatr. Orthop.* **2009**, *29*, 9–13. [CrossRef] [PubMed]
62. Wenger, D.E.; Kendell, K.R.; Miner, M.R.; Trousdale, R.T. Acetabular labral tears rarely occur in the absence of bony abnormalities. *Clin. Orthop. Relat. Res.* **2004**, *426*, 145–150. [CrossRef] [PubMed]
63. Boykin, R.E.; Anz, A.W.; Bushnell, B.D.; Kocher, M.S.; Stubbs, A.J.; Philippon, M.J. Hip instability. *J. Am. Acad. Orthop. Surg.* **2011**, *19*, 340–349. [CrossRef] [PubMed]
64. Domb, B.G.; Philippon, M.J.; Giordano, B.D. Arthroscopic capsulotomy, capsular repair, and capsular plication of the hip: Relation to atraumatic instability. *Arthroscopy* **2013**, *29*, 162–173. [CrossRef]
65. Philippon, M.J.; Stubbs, A.J.; Schenker, M.L.; Maxwell, R.B.; Ganz, R.; Leunig, M. Arthroscopic management of femoroacetabular impingement: Osteoplasty technique and literature review. *Am. J. Sport. Med.* **2007**, *35*, 1571–1580. [CrossRef]
66. Kim, K.-I.; Cho, Y.-J.; Ramteke, A.; Yoo, M.-C. Peri-acetabular rotational osteotomy with concomitant hip arthroscopy for treatment of hip dysplasia. *J. Bone Joint Surg. Br.* **2011**, *93*, 732e7. [CrossRef]
67. Leunig, M.; Siebenrock, K.A.; Ganz, R. Rationale of periacetabular osteotomy and background work. *Instr. Course Lect.* **2001**, *50*, 229–238. [CrossRef]
68. Ko, J.Y.; Wang, C.J.; Lin, C.F.; Shih, C.H. Periacetabular osteotomy through a modified Ollier transtrochanteric approach for treatment of painful dysplastic hips. *J. Bone Joint Surg. Am.* **2002**, *84*, 1594–1604. [CrossRef]
69. McCarthy, J.C.; Lee, J.A. The role of hip arthroscopy: Useful adjunct or devil's tool? *Orthopedics* **2002**, *25*, 947–948. [CrossRef]

70. Pierannunzii, L.; d'Imporzano, M. Treatment of femoroacetabular impingement: A modified resection osteoplasty technique through an anterior approach. *Orthopedics* **2007**, *30*, 96–102.
71. Robertson, W.J.; Kadrmas, W.R.; Kelly, B.T. Arthroscopic management of labral tears in the hip: A systematic review of the literature. *Clin. Orthop.* **2007**, *455*, 88–92. [CrossRef] [PubMed]
72. Becker, D.A.; Ramon, G.B. Double chevron subtrochanteric shortening derotational femoral osteotomy combined with total hip arthroplasty for the treatment of complete congenital dislocation of the hip in the adult. *J. Arthroplast.* **1995**, *10*, 313. [CrossRef] [PubMed]
73. Charnley, J.; Feagin, J.A. Low-friction arthroplasty in congenital subluxation of the hip. *Clin. Orthop.* **1973**, *91*, 98. [CrossRef] [PubMed]
74. Bruce, W.J.; Rizkallah, S.M.; Kwon, Y.M.; Goldberg, J.A.; Walsh, W.R. A new technique of subtrochanteric shortening in total hip arthroplasty: Surgical technique and results of 9 cases. *J. Arthroplast.* **2000**, *15*, 617. [CrossRef] [PubMed]
75. Cameron, H.U.; Eren, O.T.; Solomon, M. Nerve injury in the prosthetic management of the dysplastic hip. *Orthopedics* **1998**, *9*, 980. [CrossRef]
76. Chareancholvanich, K.; Beckor, D.A.; Gustilo, R.B. Treatment of congenital dislocated hip by arthroplasty with femoral shortening. *Clin. Orthop.* **1999**, *360*, 127. [CrossRef]
77. Charity, J.A.; Tsiridis, E.; Sheeraz, A.; Howell, J.R.; Hubble, M.J.W.; Timperley, A.J.; Gie, G.A. Treatment of Crowe IV high hip dysplasia with total hip replacement using the Exeter stem and shortening derotational subtrochanteric osteotomy. *J. Bone Joint Surg. Br.* **2011**, *93*, 34. [CrossRef]
78. Sponseller, P.D.; McBeath, A.A. Subtrochanteric osteotomy with intramedullary fixation for arthroplasty of the dysplastic hip: A case report. *J. Arthroplast.* **1988**, *3*, 351–354. [CrossRef]
79. Li, X.; Sun, J.; Lin, X.; Xu, S.; Tang, T. Cementless total hip arthroplasty with a double chevron subtrochanteric shortening osteotomy in patients with Crowe type-IV hip dysplasia. *Acta Orthop. Belg.* **2013**, *79*, 287.
80. Harris, W.H. Traumatic arthritis of the hip after dislocation and acetabular fractures: Treatment by mold arthroplasty. An end-result study using a new method of result evaluation. *J. Bone Joint Surg. Am.* **1969**, *51*, 737–755. [CrossRef]
81. Shapira, J.; Chen, S.L.; Rosinsky, P.J.; Maldonado, D.R.; Lall, A.C.; Domb, B.G. Outcomes of outpatient total hip arthroplasty: A systematic review. *Hip Int.* **2021**, *31*, 4–11. [CrossRef] [PubMed]
82. Healy, W.L.; Iorio, R.; Clair, A.J.; Pellegrini, V.D.; Della Valle, C.J.; Berend, K.R. Complications of Total Hip Arthroplasty: Standardized List, Definitions, and Stratification Developed by The Hip Society. *Clin. Orthop. Relat. Res.* **2016**, *474*, 357–364. [CrossRef] [PubMed]
83. Heo, S.M.; Harris, I.; Naylor, J.; Lewin, A.M. Complications to 6 months following total hip or knee arthroplasty: Observations from an Australian clinical outcomes registry. *BMC Musculoskelet. Disord.* **2020**, *21*, 602. [CrossRef] [PubMed]

**Disclaimer/Publisher's Note:** The statements, opinions and data contained in all publications are solely those of the individual author(s) and contributor(s) and not of MDPI and/or the editor(s). MDPI and/or the editor(s) disclaim responsibility for any injury to people or property resulting from any ideas, methods, instructions or products referred to in the content.

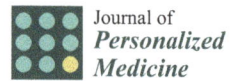

*Technical Note*

# The Deep-MCL Line: A Reliable Anatomical Landmark to Optimize the Tibial Cut in UKA

Sébastien Parratte [1,2,*], Jeremy Daxhelet [3], Jean-Noel Argenson [2] and Cécile Batailler [4,5,*]

1. Department of Orthopaedic Surgery, International Knee and Joint Centre, Hazza Bin Zayed St., Abu Dhabi P.O. Box 46705, United Arab Emirates
2. Department of Orthopedics and Traumatology, St. Marguerite Hospital, Aix Marseille University, Institute of Movement and Locomotion, 270 Bd de Sainte-Marguerite, 13009 Marseille, France; jean-noel.argenson@ap-hm.fr
3. Department of Orthopaedic Surgery, Clinique Saint-Luc Bouge, Rue Saint-Luc 8, 5004 Namur, Belgium; daxheletjeremy@gmail.com
4. Department of Orthopaedics, Croix Rousse Hospital, University of Lyon 1, 69004 Lyon, France
5. Claude Bernard Lyon 1 University, LBMC UMR_T9406, 69100 Lyon, France
* Correspondence: sebastien.parratte@gmail.com (S.P.); cecile-batailler@hotmail.fr (C.B.)

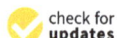

Citation: Parratte, S.; Daxhelet, J.; Argenson, J.-N.; Batailler, C. The Deep-MCL Line: A Reliable Anatomical Landmark to Optimize the Tibial Cut in UKA. *J. Pers. Med.* 2023, *13*, 855. https://doi.org/10.3390/jpm13050855

Academic Editor: Johannes Beckmann

Received: 27 March 2023
Revised: 13 May 2023
Accepted: 15 May 2023
Published: 19 May 2023

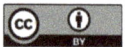

**Copyright:** © 2023 by the authors. Licensee MDPI, Basel, Switzerland. This article is an open access article distributed under the terms and conditions of the Creative Commons Attribution (CC BY) license (https://creativecommons.org/licenses/by/4.0/).

**Abstract:** The extramedullary guides for the tibial resection during medial unicompartmental knee arthroplasty (UKA) are inaccurate, with an error risk in coronal and sagittal planes and cut thickness. It was our hypothesis that the use of anatomical landmarks for the tibial cut can help the surgeon to improve accuracy. The technique described in this paper is based on the use of a simple and reproducible anatomical landmark. This landmark is the line of insertion of the fibers of the deep medial collateral ligament (MCL) around the anterior half of the medial tibial plateau called the "Deep MCL insertion line". The used anatomical landmark determines the orientation (in the coronal and sagittal planes) and the thickness of the tibial cut. This landmark corresponds to the line of insertion of the fibers of the deep MCL around the anterior half of the medial tibial plateau. A consecutive series of patients who underwent primary medial UKA between 2019 and 2021 were retrospectively reviewed. A total of 50 UKA were included. The mean age at the time of surgery was 54.5 ± 6.6 years (44–79). The radiographic measurements showed very good to excellent intra-observer and inter-observer agreements. The limb and implant alignments and the tibial positioning were satisfying, with a low rate of outliers and good restoration of the native anatomy. The landmark of the insertion of deep MCL constitutes a reliable and reproducible reference for the tibial cut axis and thickness during medial UKA, independent of the wear severity.

**Keywords:** medial unicompartmental knee arthroplasty; anatomical landmarks; coronal alignment; tibial slope; deep medial collateral ligament

## 1. Introduction

Unicompartmental knee arthroplasty (UKA) remains a demanding surgical procedure, and optimal implant positioning is essential to obtain satisfactory outcomes [1–3]. Various complications can occur after UKA, such as implant malpositioning, malalignment, and implant over- or under-sizing. Sub-optimal implant position can cause the failure of the UKA, with potential complications such as persistent pains or tibial component loosening [1–3].

As several systems use the tibial resection as a reference for the femoral resection, optimizing the tibial cut is a crucial step of the surgery. This is even more important as the risk of implant malpositioning concerns mainly the tibial implant, with a risk of outliers in the coronal and sagittal alignment and a risk of excessive tibial resection [4,5]. The extramedullary guides for the tibial resection have been improved over time, but several studies reported a persistent high percentage of outliers [5–7] with a risk of error in coronal and sagittal planes. Assistive technologies, such as robotic-assisted systems, have been developed to improve the accuracy of bone resections and implant positioning in UKA [8–10] with promising results [6,11–14]. Due to the high cost of these devices, however, less than 1% of the surgeons in the world have access to a robotic-assisted system for UKA. Therefore, it was our hypothesis that the use of simple anatomical landmarks for bone tibial bone resection can be reliable and help surgeons to improve tibial cut accuracy with conventional instrumentation. Several studies have described and assessed bony landmarks for the tibial rotation in UKA [15–17]; however, to our knowledge, no study has described the use of tibial anatomical landmarks for the orientation and the thickness of the tibial cut in medial UKA.

Therefore, the aims of this paper were as follows: (1) to describe the surgical technique of the tibial cut in UKA using the tibial insertion of the fibers of the deep medial collateral ligament (MCL) as a landmark for frontal and sagittal orientation and the thickness of resection; (2) to assess the accuracy of the tibial cut with this surgical technique as measured on post-operative radiographs (MPTA, tibial slope, joint line height, and HKA angle).

## 2. Materials and Methods

### 2.1. Surgical Technique

The medial UKA is indicated for osteoarthritis without severe constitutional deformity. The UKA principles are to compensate for the wear, respect the anatomy of the proximal tibial epiphysis, and perform a pure resurfacing surgery, respecting the ligamentous envelope. Based on the literature, angular limits of resection can be comprised between 0 and 5 degrees of varus for the frontal plane and between 2 and 6 degrees of posterior slope for the sagittal plane. Following the standard surgical technique, the tibial cut is performed using a conventional extramedullary guide, the surgeon aiming for the ideal position of the jig to reach the goals of resection in terms of thickness of resection and frontal/sagittal orientation based on its own judgment (Figure 1). Fine adjustments of the cut axis can be challenging, and this might explain the degrees of inaccuracy observed with conventional instrumentation in the literature.

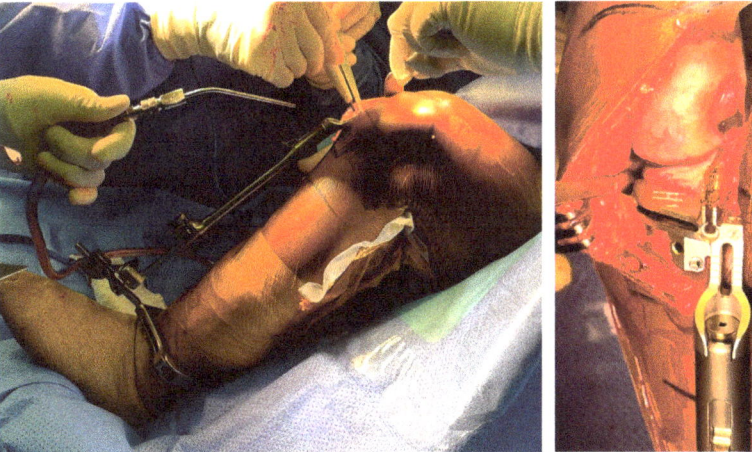

**Figure 1.** Extramedullary guide to check the tibial slope and the coronal axis for the tibial cut.

The technique described in this paper is based on the use of a simple and reproducible anatomical landmark. This landmark is the line of insertion of the fibers of the deep MCL around the anterior half of the medial tibial plateau called the "Deep MCL insertion line". The visualization of this line is relatively simple when performing a very conservative approach exposure (without any release of the medial tibial plateau) and after the removal of the anterior osteophytes. For this technique, two points are marked along the insertion of the deep MCL, and then the line joining these two points is drawn on the bone using the electrocautery knife. The used anatomical landmark determines the orientation (in the coronal and sagittal planes) and the thickness of the tibial cut. The cutting jig can then be directly aligned onto this line and pinned, the lower part of the jig being used only as a support of the cutting jig. A second check can be performed once the cutting jig is set up.

A medial subvastus approach without any medial or lateral release is performed. The deep MCL insertion is visualized, and two points (one anterior and one more posterior) are marked along its insertion around the anterior part of the medial tibial plateau (Figure 2a). These two points are used to draw a line which is usually just below the medial osteophytes. These medial osteophytes can be partially removed to better visualize the insertion of the fibers around the tibial plateau if needed (Figure 2b). To remove these osteophytes while avoiding any damage to the MCL insertion, a small Hohmann retractor can be used. Following the line of the MCL insertion around the medial tibial plateau and extending this line anteriorly can accurately guide the frontal and sagittal orientation of the cut (posterior slope) and the thickness of resection. Indeed, the medial osteophyte is frequently used as a landmark medially but shows only the thickness of the cut medially and anteriorly. It is thus insufficient to avoid a valgus cut compared to the line that has been described earlier (Figure 3). As the level of the insertion of the deep MCL is fixed and not related to the severity of the wear or osteoarthritis, this landmark can reliably be used to determine the thickness of the cut. The use of a tibial stylus, whose size varies significantly with the severity of the wear, is thus not necessary. The tibial rotation is determined as usual, drawing a line between the point considered the medial point to the tibial insertion of the anterior cruciate ligament and the most anterior point of the medial tibial plateau. This line is parallel to the lateral facet of the medial condyle.

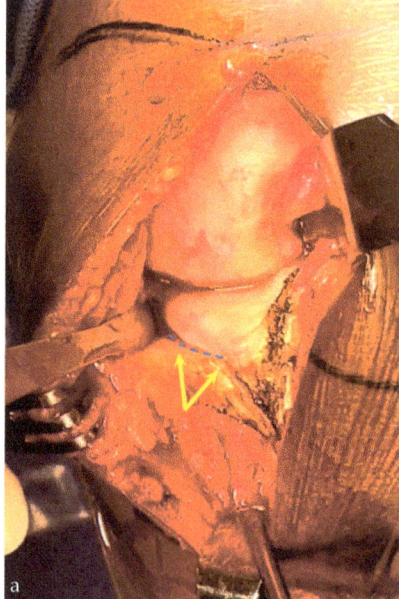 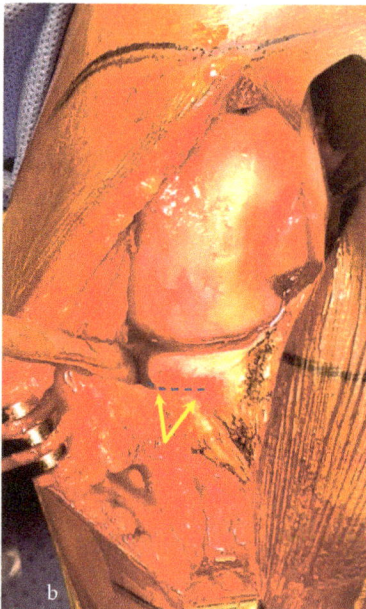

**Figure 2.** Insertion of the deep medial collateral ligament (MCL) on the medial proximal tibial plateau (yellow arrows), which delineates the tibial cut axis (blue line) (**a**). The osteophytes resection improves the visualization of this landmark (**b**).

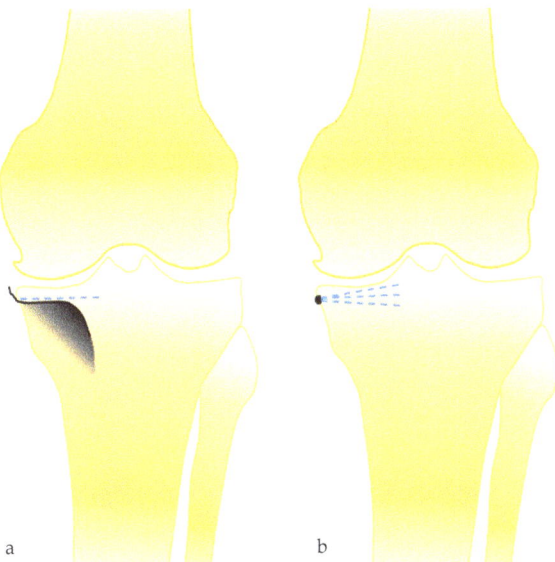

**Figure 3.** The deep MCL landmark allows us to determine the coronal axis of the tibial cut (**a**), and not only the height of the tibial cut medially, as the medial osteophyte landmark (**b**).

When the cutting guide can be positioned on the desired cut axis and set in place (Figure 4). The tibial cut is performed with the saw as usual. To confirm the cut axis and thickness, the tibial resection should have almost no attachment with the articular capsule (cut inside the ligamentous envelope) (Figure 5). The final implant is positioned in the ligamentous envelope, preserving the deep MCL insertion and the joint line height. The meniscal scar was used to evaluate the restoration of the joint line, the upper level of the polyethylene insert being exactly at the level of the meniscal scar (Figure 6).

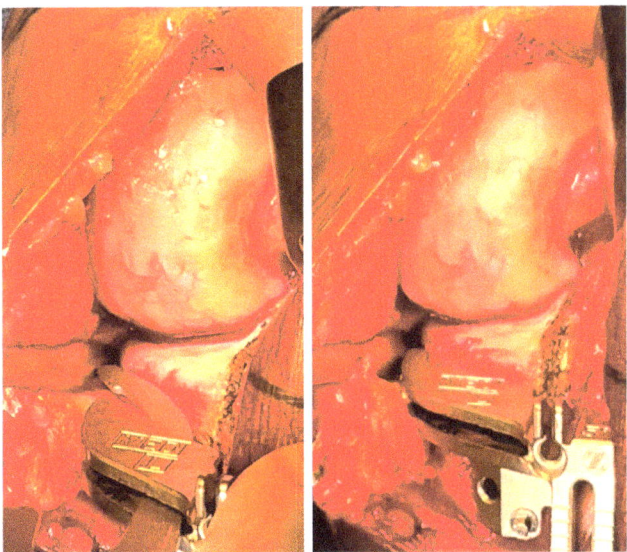

**Figure 4.** After the visualization of the tibial landmark, the cutting guide is positioned directly on this landmark and then set to the bone.

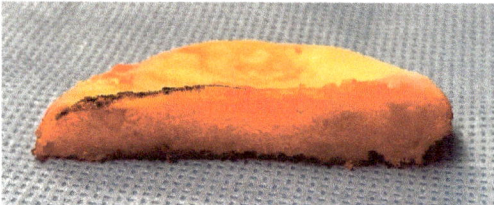
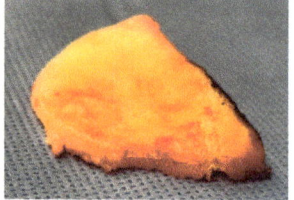

**Figure 5.** The tibial resection allows to confirm if the cut axis is satisfying: the cut tightness should be similar anteriorly and posteriorly, and the cut should be at the limit of the capsular attaches.

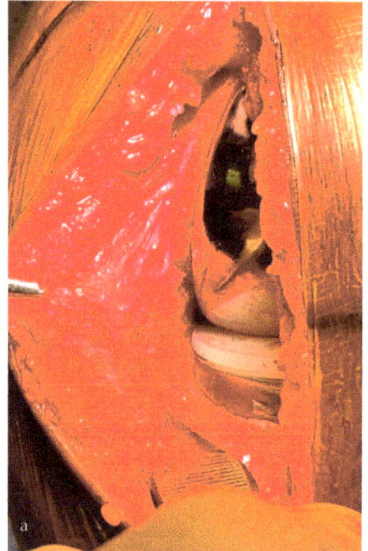
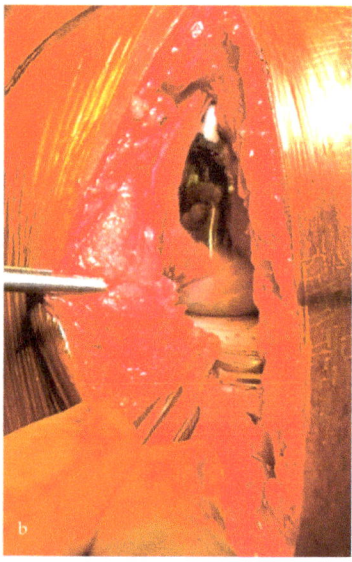

**Figure 6.** With the definitive implants, the tibial implant should be positioned in the soft tissues' envelope respecting the deep MCL (**a**) and restoring the joint line height, visualized with the meniscal scar level (**b**).

*2.2. Patients*

After obtaining ethics internal review board approval, a consecutive series of patients who underwent a primary medial UKA between 2019 and 2021 at a single institution were retrospectively reviewed. The indication for surgery was medial femorotibial osteoarthritis or femoral osteonecrosis, with a reducible deformation and without anterior laxity. Exclusion criteria were incomplete data (radiographs) and previous tibial osteotomy. Of the 59 primary UKA performed during this period, 50 met the criteria (6 lateral UKA and 3 patients with incomplete radiographs). The mean age at the time of surgery was $54.5 \pm 6.6$ years (44–79). Mean BMI was $32.7 \pm 3.7$ kg/m$^2$ (27–44). A total of 40% ($n = 20$) were male patients, and 48% ($n = 24$) were operated on the left knee. A total of 24% had a grade 4, and 76% had a grade 3 of medial femorotibial osteoarthritis (Kellgren Lawrence). All UKA were performed using conventional instrumentation by a single senior surgeon with 15 years of experience in UKA. All patients received the same cemented morphometric fixed-bearing medial UKA (Persona Partial Knee System, Zimmer Biomet, Warsaw, IN, USA) [18]. This system is a tibia-based technique using the spacer-block technique for femoral preparation [18,19]. The tibial cut is thus an essential factor in the quality of the distal femoral cut and the entire procedure.

## 2.3. Data Assessment

The radiographic assessment was performed preoperatively and at 2 months, including an anteroposterior view, lateral view of the knee, and a long-leg standing radiograph performed according to a standardized protocol in the same radiological center. Standardized radiographic measurements were performed: HKA angle, mechanical Medial Distal Femoral Angle (mMDFA), Medial Proximal Tibial Angle (MPTA), tibial slope, the joint line height, the Cartier angle, the coronal axis, and the thickness of the tibial cut. Restitution of joint line height was assessed using the two methods of Weber [20]. The tibial resection was measured with the technique described by Negrin [21]. The radiographs were calibrated, allowing an accurate measurement up to 0.1 mm. Radiological measurements were performed twice by two independent reviewers (CB and JD) for all measurements to assess the reliability of each measurement. The thickness of the polyethylene insert was reported in the surgical report.

## 2.4. Statistical Analysis

Statistical analysis was performed using the XL STAT software (Version 2021.2.1, Addinsoft Inc., Paris, France). Data were described using means, standard deviation, ranges for continuous variables, and counts (percent) for categorical variables. The intra- and inter-observer reliabilities of the radiographic measurements were evaluated by an intraclass correlation coefficient. Strength of agreement for the kappa coefficient was interpreted as follows: <0.20 = unacceptable, 0.20–0.39 = questionable, 0.40–0.59 = good, 0.60–0.79 = very good, and 0.80–1 = excellent [22].

## 3. Results

The radiographic measurements showed very good to excellent intra-observer and inter-observer agreements (Table 1). The limb and implant alignments and the tibial positioning are reported in Table 2. The tibial insert was 8 mm for 50% of the patients ($n$ = 25), 9 mm for 48% ($n$ = 24), and 10 mm for 2% ($n$ = 1).

**Table 1.** Intraobserver and interobserver coefficients for the radiographic measurement.

|  | Intra Observer ICC | Inter Observer ICC | Agreement |
|---|---|---|---|
| HKA angle | 0.98 | 0.98 | Excellent |
| mMDFA | 0.95 | 0.92 | Excellent |
| MPTA | 0.90 | 0.83 | Excellent |
| Tibial slope | 0.82 | 0.83 | Excellent |
| Cartier angle | 0.85 | 0.69 | Very good |
| Joint line height | 0.85 | 0.72 | Very good |
| Tibial cut height | 0.80 | 0.75 | Very good |
| Tibial cut Coronal Axis | 0.87 | 0.78 | Very good |

Strength of agreement for the kappa coefficient was interpreted as follows: <0.20 = unacceptable, 0.20–0.39 = questionable, 0.40–0.59 = good, 0.60–0.79 = very good, and 0.80–1 = excellent.

**Table 2.** Preoperative and postoperative radiographic measurements and outliers.

|  | Preoperative Data N = 50 | Postoperative Data N = 50 |
|---|---|---|
| HKA (°) (mean ± SD) [Min; Max] | 173.5 ± 3.6 [164.6; 180] | 176.5 ± 3.1 [170; 185] |
| mMDFA (°) (mean ± SD) [Min; Max] | 91.2 ± 2.2 [87; 96] | 92.2 ± 2.3 [88; 96] |
| MPTA (°) (mean ± SD) [Min; Max] OUTLIERS MPTA < 85° | 86.4 ± 1.5 [83; 89] 6 (12%) | 86.8 ± 1.5 [84; 90] 1 (2%) |

**Table 2.** *Cont.*

|  | Preoperative Data N = 50 | Postoperative Data N = 50 |
|---|---|---|
| Slope (°) (mean ± SD) [Min; Max] OUTLIERS Slope < 78° | 80.9 ± 3.2 [74; 87] 7 (14%) | 82.6 ± 2.3 [78; 87] 0 |
| Cartier angle (°) (mean ± SD) [Min; Max] | 2.6 ± 2.8 [−3; 7] | - - |
| Joint line height (femoral cortex) (mm) (mean ± SD) [Min; Max] | - | 0.9 ± 1.1 [−1.7; 4.5] |
| Joint line height (femoral diaphysis) (mm) (mean ± SD) [Min; Max] OUTLIERS Joint line height > 2 mm | - | 0.8 ± 1.1 [−1.7; 4.5] 3 (6%) |
| Tibial resection height (mm) (mean ± SD) [Min; Max] | - | 6.0 ± 1.7 [1; 9.5] |
| Tibial cut axis (°) (mean ± SD) [Min; Max] OUTLIERS Tibial cut axis < 85° OUTLIERS Tibial cut axis > 90° | - | 87.7 ± 1.6 [84; 92] 1 (2%) 2 (4%) |
| Difference between tibial cut and Cartier angle (°) (mean in absolute value ± SD) [Min; Max] | - | 0.57 ± 1.1 [−5; 4] |

HKA: Hip Knee Ankle angle; mMDFA: mechanical Medial Distal Femoral Angle; MPTA: Medial Proximal Tibial Angle; JLCA: Joint Line Convergence Angle; JLO: Joint Line Orientation; SD: Standard Deviation.

## 4. Discussion

The tibial cut is a challenging step during medial UKA. This surgical technique based on a bony landmark aims to reduce the error risk of the tibial cut axis. This technique was performed for many years by the senior surgeon with satisfying results and appears safe and reliable.

Several limitations should be outlined in our study. This study was not comparative with other surgical techniques (robotic-assisted or manual with extramedullary guide). There were no functional outcomes or long-term data. Nevertheless, this study aimed to describe for the first time the surgical technique of the tibial cut in UKA using the tibial insertion of the fibers of the deep MCL and its accuracy. A long-term comparative study would be interesting to perform secondarily.

Tibial malpositioning is one of the most common errors during medial UKA [6]. The risk is to perform the tibial cut in the valgus or varus compared to the epiphyseal axis. The mean axis of the tibial cut was satisfying in this study (87.7° ± 1.6°), with only one patient with a tibial cut axis superior to 5° of varus (84°). The mean difference between the tibial cut axis and the tibial epiphyseal axis was inferior to 0.6° ± 1.1. Two main philosophies for positioning UKA components are described in the literature [23]. The mechanical alignment technique references the mechanical axis of long bones and makes frontal bone cuts perpendicular to them [24]. This technique is easier to perform than the conventional technique because the tibial cut is performed at 90° of the tibial mechanical axes. An alternative alignment technique was popularized by Cartier who tried to reproduce the tibial epiphyseal axis with the tibial cut in the coronal plane [25,26]. A threshold value is recommended with a tibial cut inferior to 5° of varus compared to the tibial mechanical axis. This last philosophy avoids a valgus cut compared to the epiphyseal axis with a risk of loosening or secondary subsidence due to the soft bone in the lateral part of the tibial resection [23]. To reproduce the tibial epiphyseal anatomy also aims to obtain a perfect congruence between the femoral implant and the plateau surface and avoid a position on the edges of the condylar implant. However, to perform a tibial cut with some degree of varus with an extramedullary guide is difficult and inaccurate. The rate of outliers in the coronal plane after conventional medial UKA is significant in the literature up to 35% [4,6]. To limit the number of outliers in UKA, robotic surgery has been developed, but its access remains limited to only a subset of surgeons, and its cost-efficiency is still to be demonstrated. The landmark described in this study is a simple, cost-efficient additional control to improve the accuracy of the tibial resection and reduce the number of outliers. The advantage of this technique compared to the medial osteophyte landmark is the line following the insertion of deep MCL determines the coronal and sagittal planes (Figure 3). The quality of the tibial cut also determines the femoral implant positioning. Most of the UKA surgical techniques have femoral cuts dependent on the tibial cut. If the alignment of the tibial cut is not satisfying, the femoral implant has a risk of malpositioning.

In this study, the joint line height was distalized at a mean of 0.9 mm ± 1.1 compared to the pre-operative X-rays, probably due to the pre-operative wear of the femoral condyle. Taking this point into consideration, the restitution of the joint line height using this tibial landmark was thus satisfying with the smallest insert sizes (8 or 9 mm). Restitution of joint line height after UKA, and particularly avoidance of excessive tibial resection, has a major impact on patients' outcomes and tibial implant survivorship [27–29]. In addition to making the tibial implant rest on more fragile cancellous bone, excessive tibial cutting also leads to shifting the contact point of the femoral component towards the periphery of the tibial plateau due to the plateau's funnel shape. A biomechanical study demonstrated that after UKA, the mean strain on the proximal tibial cortex increased by 6%, 13%, and 18% when tibial resection levels of 2 mm, 4 mm, and 6 mm were modeled, respectively [29]. Another study demonstrated similar results: 4 mm increased distal resection increased tibial strain variance by 35% [27]. An excessive tibial cut can also lead to a distalization of the femoral implant by dependent cuts, lower the joint line height in the medial compartment, and result in a no-anatomical oblique joint line [26]. The improvement of the joint line height can reduce the polyethylene wear, the loosening risk, and the progression of osteoarthritis in the contralateral compartment [1,30]. A reduction in tibial resection may also improve some tibial pain due to the excessive strain on the proximal tibial cortex [27]. The landmark of the insertion of deep MCL constitutes a stable reference for the cut thickness, independent of the wear severity and the position of the tibial sizer. This landmark can increase the reproducibility of the tibial resection, and this might be particularly helpful and cost-efficient for surgeons with a low volume of UKA.

## 5. Conclusions

The results of our study confirmed that the deep-MCL line is a reliable anatomical landmark to optimize the tibial cut in UKA. This landmark corresponds to the line of insertion of the fibers of the deep MCL around the anterior half of the medial tibial plateau. The deep-MCL line can help surgeons to improve the accuracy and the reproducibility of the tibial cut in UKA for both the coronal and the sagittal plans. This technique can help to reduce the outliers without the extra cost related to the use of assistive computer-assisted technologies.

**Author Contributions:** Conceptualization, S.P., J.-N.A. and C.B.; methodology, S.P. and C.B.; validation, S.P., J.D., J.-N.A. and C.B.; formal analysis, J.D. and C.B.; data curation, J.D. and C.B.; writing—original draft preparation, S.P. and C.B.; writing—review and editing, J.D. and J.-N.A.; supervision, S.P. All authors have read and agreed to the published version of the manuscript.

**Funding:** This research received no external funding.

**Institutional Review Board Statement:** This study was approved by our hospital's Institutional Review Board (study ID Number: MF3867, approval date: 20 December 2020). All procedures were performed in accordance with the ethical standards of the institutional and/or national research committee, the 1964 Helsinki declaration, and its later amendments, or comparable ethical standards.

**Informed Consent Statement:** Informed consent was obtained from all subjects involved in this study.

**Data Availability Statement:** Data is unavailable due to ethical restrictions.

**Conflicts of Interest:** The authors declare no conflict of interest related to this work. S.P.: Royalties from Zimmer Biomet and Newclip; Consultant for Zimmer Biomet; Treasurer for European Knee Society. J.D. and C.B.: No conflict of interest. J.-N.A.: Educational Consultant and royalties from Zimmer-Biomet.

## References

1. Barbadoro, P.; Ensini, A.; Leardini, A.; d'Amato, M.; Feliciangeli, A.; Timoncini, A.; Amadei, F.; Belvedere, C.; Giannini, S. Tibial component alignment and risk of loosening in unicompartmental knee arthroplasty: A radiographic and radiostereometric study. *Knee Surg. Sport. Traumatol. Arthrosc.* **2014**, *22*, 3157–3162. [CrossRef]
2. Epinette, J.A.; Brunschweiler, B.; Mertl, P.; Mole, D.; Cazenave, A.; The French Society for the Hip and Knee. Unicompartmental knee arthroplasty modes of failure: Wear is not the main reason for failure: A multicentre study of 418 failed knees. *Orthop. Traumatol. Surg. Res.* **2012**, *98*, S124–S130. [CrossRef]
3. Ko, Y.B.; Gujarathi, M.R.; Oh, K.J. Outcome of Unicompartmental Knee Arthroplasty: A Systematic Review of Comparative Studies between Fixed and Mobile Bearings Focusing on Complications. *Knee Surg. Relat. Res.* **2015**, *27*, 141–148. [CrossRef]
4. Bell, S.W.; Anthony, I.; Jones, B.; MacLean, A.; Rowe, P.; Blyth, M. Improved Accuracy of Component Positioning with Robotic-Assisted Unicompartmental Knee Arthroplasty: Data from a Prospective, Randomized Controlled Study. *J. Bone Jt. Surg. Am. Vol.* **2016**, *98*, 627–635. [CrossRef] [PubMed]
5. Ponzio, D.Y.; Lonner, J.H. Robotic Technology Produces More Conservative Tibial Resection Than Conventional Techniques in UKA. *Am. J. Orthop.* **2016**, *45*, E465–E468.
6. Batailler, C.; White, N.; Ranaldi, F.M.; Neyret, P.; Servien, E.; Lustig, S. Improved implant position and lower revision rate with robotic-assisted unicompartmental knee arthroplasty. *Knee Surg. Sport. Traumatol. Arthrosc.* **2019**, *27*, 1232–1240. [CrossRef]
7. Herry, Y.; Batailler, C.; Lording, T.; Servien, E.; Neyret, P.; Lustig, S. Improved joint-line restitution in unicompartmental knee arthroplasty using a robotic-assisted surgical technique. *Int. Orthop.* **2017**, *41*, 2265–2271. [CrossRef]
8. Thilak, J.; Thadi, M.; Mane, P.P.; Sharma, A.; Mohan, V.; Babu, B.C. Accuracy of tibial component positioning in the robotic arm assisted versus conventional unicompartmental knee arthroplasty. *J. Orthop.* **2020**, *22*, 367–371. [CrossRef]
9. Gaudiani, M.A.; Nwachukwu, B.U.; Baviskar, J.V.; Sharma, M.; Ranawat, A.S. Optimization of sagittal and coronal planes with robotic-assisted unicompartmental knee arthroplasty. *Knee* **2017**, *24*, 837–843. [CrossRef] [PubMed]
10. Savov, P.; Tuecking, L.R.; Windhagen, H.; Calliess, T.; Ettinger, M. Robotics improves alignment accuracy and reduces early revision rates for UKA in the hands of low-volume UKA surgeons. *Arch. Orthop. Trauma. Surg.* **2021**, *141*, 2139–2146. [CrossRef] [PubMed]
11. Robinson, P.G.; Clement, N.D.; Hamilton, D.; Blyth, M.J.G.; Haddad, F.S.; Patton, J.T. A systematic review of robotic-assisted unicompartmental knee arthroplasty: Prosthesis design and type should be reported. *Bone Jt. J.* **2019**, *101*, 838–847. [CrossRef]
12. Kayani, B.; Haddad, F.S. Robotic unicompartmental knee arthroplasty: Current challenges and future perspectives. *Bone Jt. Res.* **2019**, *8*, 228–231. [CrossRef]
13. Zambianchi, F.; Daffara, V.; Franceschi, G.; Banchelli, F.; Marcovigi, A.; Catani, F. Robotic arm-assisted unicompartmental knee arthroplasty: High survivorship and good patient-related outcomes at a minimum five years of follow-up. *Knee Surg. Sport. Traumatol. Arthrosc.* **2021**, *29*, 3316–3322. [CrossRef] [PubMed]
14. Gilmour, A.; MacLean, A.D.; Rowe, P.J.; Banger, M.S.; Donnelly, I.; Jones, B.G.; Blyth, M.J.G. Robotic-Arm-Assisted vs. Conventional Unicompartmental Knee Arthroplasty. The 2-Year Clinical Outcomes of a Randomized Controlled Trial. *J. Arthroplast.* **2018**, *33*, S109–S115. [CrossRef] [PubMed]
15. Kawahara, S.; Matsuda, S.; Okazaki, K.; Tashiro, Y.; Iwamoto, Y. Is the medial wall of the intercondylar notch useful for tibial rotational reference in unicompartmental knee arthroplasty? *Clin. Orthop. Relat. Res.* **2012**, *470*, 1177–1184. [CrossRef]
16. Lee, S.Y.; Chay, S.; Lim, H.C.; Bae, J.H. Tibial component rotation during the unicompartmental knee arthroplasty: Is the anterior superior iliac spine an appropriate landmark? *Knee Surg. Sport. Traumatol. Arthrosc.* **2017**, *25*, 3723–3732. [CrossRef]
17. Makhdom, A.M.; Kerr, G.J.; Wu, E.; Lonner, J.H. Rotational alignment errors can occur in unicompartmental knee arthroplasty if anatomical landmarks are misused: A preoperative CT scan analysis. *Knee* **2020**, *27*, 242–248. [CrossRef]
18. Parratte, S.; Sah, A.; Batailler, C. Safe and reliable clinical outcomes at 2 years of a fixed-bearing partial knee arthroplasty with a morphometric tibial tray in a large worldwide population. *Knee Surg. Sport. Traumatol. Arthrosc.* **2023**, *31*, 814–821. [CrossRef]
19. National Joint Registry for England and Wales: 17th Annual Report. 2020. Available online: https://reports.njrcentre.org.uk/Portals/0/PDFdownloads/NJR%2017th%20Annual%20Report%202020.pdf (accessed on 14 May 2023).
20. Weber, P.; Schroder, C.; Laubender, R.P.; Baur-Melnyk, A.; von Schulze Pellengahr, C.; Jansson, V.; Muller, P.E. Joint line reconstruction in medial unicompartmental knee arthroplasty: Development and validation of a measurement method. *Knee Surg. Sport. Traumatol. Arthrosc. Off. J. ESSKA* **2013**, *21*, 2468–2473. [CrossRef]
21. Negrin, R.; Duboy, J.; Reyes, N.O.; Barahona, M.; Iniguez, M.; Infante, C.; Cordero, J.A.; Sepulveda, V.; Ferrer, G. Robotic-assisted Unicompartmental knee Arthroplasty optimizes joint line restitution better than conventional surgery. *J. Exp. Orthop.* **2020**, *7*, 94. [CrossRef] [PubMed]
22. Regier, D.A.; Narrow, W.E.; Clarke, D.E.; Kraemer, H.C.; Kuramoto, S.J.; Kuhl, E.A.; Kupfer, D.J. DSM-5 field trials in the United States and Canada, Part II: Test-retest reliability of selected categorical diagnoses. *Am. J. Psychiatry* **2013**, *170*, 59–70. [CrossRef] [PubMed]

23. Riviere, C.; Sivaloganathan, S.; Villet, L.; Cartier, P.; Lustig, S.; Vendittoli, P.A.; Cobb, J. Kinematic alignment of medial UKA is safe: A systematic review. *Knee Surg. Sport. Traumatol. Arthrosc.* **2021**, *30*, 1082–1094. [CrossRef] [PubMed]
24. Walker, T.; Heinemann, P.; Bruckner, T.; Streit, M.R.; Kinkel, S.; Gotterbarm, T. The influence of different sets of surgical instrumentation in Oxford UKA on bearing size and component position. *Arch. Orthop. Trauma. Surg.* **2017**, *137*, 895–902. [CrossRef] [PubMed]
25. Bonnin, M.; Chambat, P. Current status of valgus angle, tibial head closing wedge osteotomy in media gonarthrosis. *Orthopade* **2004**, *33*, 135–142. [CrossRef]
26. Deschamps, G.; Chol, C. Fixed-bearing unicompartmental knee arthroplasty. Patients' selection and operative technique. *Orthop. Traumatol. Surg. Res. OTSR* **2011**, *97*, 648–661. [CrossRef]
27. Small, S.R.; Berend, M.E.; Rogge, R.D.; Archer, D.B.; Kingman, A.L.; Ritter, M.A. Tibial loading after UKA: Evaluation of tibial slope, resection depth, medial shift and component rotation. *J. Arthroplast.* **2013**, *28*, 179–183. [CrossRef]
28. Kwon, O.R.; Kang, K.T.; Son, J.; Suh, D.S.; Baek, C.; Koh, Y.G. Importance of joint line preservation in unicompartmental knee arthroplasty: Finite element analysis. *J. Orthop. Res. Off. Publ. Orthop. Res. Soc.* **2017**, *35*, 347–352. [CrossRef]
29. Simpson, D.J.; Price, A.J.; Gulati, A.; Murray, D.W.; Gill, H.S. Elevated proximal tibial strains following unicompartmental knee replacement–a possible cause of pain. *Med. Eng. Phys.* **2009**, *31*, 752–757. [CrossRef]
30. Collier, M.B.; Eickmann, T.H.; Sukezaki, F.; McAuley, J.P.; Engh, G.A. Patient, implant, and alignment factors associated with revision of medial compartment unicondylar arthroplasty. *J. Arthroplast.* **2006**, *21*, 108–115. [CrossRef]

**Disclaimer/Publisher's Note:** The statements, opinions and data contained in all publications are solely those of the individual author(s) and contributor(s) and not of MDPI and/or the editor(s). MDPI and/or the editor(s) disclaim responsibility for any injury to people or property resulting from any ideas, methods, instructions or products referred to in the content.

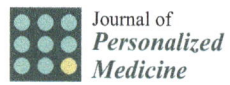 

Article

# Digital Rehabilitation after Knee Arthroplasty: A Multi-Center Prospective Longitudinal Cohort Study

Julien Lebleu [1,*], Andries Pauwels [1], Philippe Anract [2], Sébastien Parratte [3,4], Philippe Van Overschelde [5] and Stefaan Van Onsem [6,7]

1. moveUP, Cantersteen 47, 1000 Brussels, Belgium
2. Service de Chirurgie Orthopédique, Hopital Cochin, 75679 Paris, France
3. International Knee and Joint Centre, Abu Dhabi 46705, United Arab Emirates
4. Locomotion Institute, Aix Marseille University, 13009 Marseille, France
5. Hip and Knee Clinic, 9830 Gent, Belgium
6. Orthopaedics Department, AZ Alma Eeklo, Ringlaan 15, 9900 Eeklo, Belgium
7. Department of Human Structure and Repair, Ghent University, 9000 Gent, Belgium
* Correspondence: julien@moveup.care

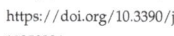

**Abstract:** Rehabilitation for total knee replacement (TKA) often involves in-person therapy sessions, which can be time consuming and costly. Digital rehabilitation has the potential to address these limitations, but most of these systems offer standardized protocols without considering the patient's pain, participation, and speed of recovery. Furthermore, most digital systems lack human support in case of need. The aim of this study was to investigate the engagement, safety, and clinical effectiveness of a personalized and adaptative app-based human-supported digital monitoring and rehabilitation program. In this prospective multi-center longitudinal cohort study, 127 patients were included. Undesired events were managed through a smart alert system. Doctors were triggered when there was a suspicion of problems. The drop-out rate, complications and readmissions, PROMS, and satisfaction were collected through the app. There was only 2% readmission. Doctor actions through the platform potentially avoided 57 consultations (85% of alerts). The adherence to the program was 77%, and 89% of the patients would recommend the use of the program. Personalized human-backed-up digital solutions can help to improve the rehabilitation journey of patients after TKA, lower healthcare-related costs by lowering the complication and readmission rate, and improve patient reported outcomes.

**Keywords:** total knee arthroplasty; knee; digital rehabilitation; telerehabilitation; mhealth; individualized

Citation: Lebleu, J.; Pauwels, A.; Anract, P.; Parratte, S.; Van Overschelde, P.; Van Onsem, S. Digital Rehabilitation after Knee Arthroplasty: A Multi-Center Prospective Longitudinal Cohort Study. *J. Pers. Med.* **2023**, *13*, 824. https://doi.org/10.3390/jpm 13050824

Academic Editor: Johannes Beckmann

Received: 7 April 2023
Revised: 9 May 2023
Accepted: 11 May 2023
Published: 13 May 2023

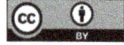

**Copyright:** © 2023 by the authors. Licensee MDPI, Basel, Switzerland. This article is an open access article distributed under the terms and conditions of the Creative Commons Attribution (CC BY) license (https:// creativecommons.org/licenses/by/ 4.0/).

## 1. Introduction

Total knee arthroplasty (TKA) is a commonly performed procedure to relieve pain and improve function in individuals with degenerative knee joint disorders [1]. Not only the number of procedures but also the cost associated with these surgeries is rising, making it important to find ways to monitor the postoperative trajectory and complications effectively [2].

Rehabilitation is a crucial component of postoperative care, as it can decrease pain, and improve function and activities of daily living [3]. However, traditional rehabilitation for total knee replacement patients often involves in-person therapy sessions, which can be time consuming and costly. In addition, adherence to home exercise therapy is often low, which can lead to suboptimal outcomes and increased healthcare costs [4,5]. The lack of access to rehabilitation services in remote and underserved areas can also be a barrier to effective rehabilitation [6].

Digital rehabilitation has the potential to address the limitations of traditional rehabilitation. Mobile apps and other technology-based tools provide individuals with access to rehabilitation therapy outside of traditional settings, which can increase engagement and improve adherence to therapy [7]. Digital rehabilitation also has the potential to increase access to rehabilitation services [8]. In addition, digital rehabilitation can provide real-time data and feedback on therapy progress, which can improve outcomes and enhance the overall rehabilitation experience. While the heterogeneity between digital rehabilitation systems and the lack of clear evidence regarding their effectiveness and safety need to be considered, digital rehabilitation holds great promise as a solution to enhance rehabilitation outcomes for total knee replacement patients [9–11]. The latest evidence on digital rehabilitation has demonstrated that it is non-inferior to face-to-face interventions and has the potential to improve outcomes for patients [12]. The growing interest in digital rehabilitation is reflected in multiple studies on telemedicine and arthroplasty in the last 5 years. This is especially true after the pandemic, as patients are looking for alternatives to traditional rehabilitation methods. Most of these systems are limited because they offer the same protocols for every patient without considering the patient's pain, participation, and speed of recovery. Furthermore, most of the available systems are not backed up by human support in case of need.

Understanding the potential of digital rehabilitation better might help to enhance the development of personalized effective rehabilitation programs for patients undergoing knee replacement surgery, and consecutively optimize patients' episode of care and outcomes. The aim of this study was to investigate the engagement, safety, clinical effectiveness, and satisfaction of a personalized and adaptative app-based human-backed-up digital monitoring, pain management, and rehabilitation program after knee replacement arthroplasty.

## 2. Materials and Methods

This interventional, multi-center, single-arm, prospective study was performed on 127 individuals with degenerative knee pain who utilized digital rehabilitation following TKA between January 2021 and May 2022. These patients underwent no face-to-face rehabilitation. Subjects were included in 1 French and 13 Belgian hospitals. Characteristics of participants are displayed in Table 1.

**Table 1.** Characteristics of study participants.

| Characteristic | Cohort ($n = 127$) |
|---|---|
| Age (years), mean (SD) | 62 (9) |
| Gender (%) | |
| *Female* | 51 |
| *Male* | 49 |
| BMI, mean (SD) | 31 (5) |

SD = standard deviation.

Individuals were invited to download an app-based telerehabilitation system.

The application 'moveUP Therapy' (moveUP®, Bruxelles, Belgium) is registered as a medical device and uses a smart virtual platform for digital rehabilitation based on objective and subjective patient data, combined with personalized interaction between a therapist and the patient. The treatment is continuously adapted and personalized automatically and clinically according to the patient's needs.

The exclusion criteria were as follows: having any preoperative (e.g., epidural catheter, urethral catheter, intra-articular catheter) or postoperative procedure that might interfere with the rehabilitation during and after hospitalization; or having any significant medical condition (e.g., Parkinson's disease, multiple sclerosis, cerebral vascular accident) or psychiatric disorder (active alcohol/drug abuse, etc.) that might interfere with the rehabilitation.

The intervention was a home-based digital intervention of exercise and education. Patients were monitored remotely by a physical therapist through a secured chat messaging system. The system is composed of a mobile app for the patient and a web-based portal that allows the physical therapist to look at patient data (physical activity, pain levels, medication use, exercise adherence, PROMS, pictures, videos) daily and to personalize the protocol accordingly. Objective data was collected throughout the recovery using a commercial activity tracker (Garmin Vivofit 4) worn 24/7 by the patients.

Based on the patient objective and subjective daily feedback, exercises were delivered daily, and patient-reported adherence was assessed for each of them, allowing the calculation of an adherence rate (ratio of exercises achieved/exercises given). The patient was asked to answer questions daily, and to record video of their knee range of motion weekly from the day of surgery until two months after surgery. If needed, the patients were also able to take pictures of the wound or the leg and share them through the app for appropriate adaptation of the treatment plan without any systematic physical consultation if not needed based on the picture analysis.

The educational component was delivered through educational articles at specific time points of the treatment. Pain management strategies such as activities or medication counseling were personalized based on the pain and activity data of the patient.

Undesired events were managed through a smart alert system. Doctors were triggered in case of suspicion of problems. The problems were raised directly by the patients, via data-based alerts, or by the physical therapist supervising the patient's status daily.

The ethics committee of the Universitair Ziekenhuis Antwerpen approved the study protocol, and each patient provided written informed consent to the use of their anonymized data for scientific use.

### 2.1. Outcomes

The drop-out rate and their reasons, complications, unplanned consultations, and readmissions were collected through the app.

Active knee range of motion was assessed by the physical therapist based on videos sent by the patients. Patients were requested to lie on a flat surface and bend the affected knee as far as possible by sliding the foot towards the buttocks, without forcing. It is important to note that there is a systematic error of almost 10° compared with range of motion measured by a clinician with a goniometer [13].

Patient-reported outcomes such as the Oxford Knee Score, Knee Osteoarthritis Outcome score (KOOS), and EuroQol 5-Dimension (EQ5D) were measured before surgery and 6 weeks, 3 months, and 6 months after surgery through the app. Satisfaction was assessed using the Knee Society Score (KSS) satisfaction scale. Furthermore, a binary satisfaction question was asked: "Would you chose digital rehabilitation again?"

The quality-adjusted life year (QALY) is a health outcome measure of disease burden that combines quality and length of life [14]. One year in perfect health equals 1 QALY, and 0 represents death. To calculate the QALY gain after surgery for our cohort, we used the EuroQol 5-Dimension (EQ-5D) and the Belgian value set [15].

### 2.2. Cost–Consequence Analysis

A cost–consequence analysis approach was chosen as no comparative analysis was possible given the absence of a control group. Cost–consequence analysis is considered a logical first step towards a formal economic evaluation [16–18]. Direct costs were analyzed separately from outcomes. Indirect cost/benefits for patients (travel time reduction) were not considered.

The per-person cost of the digital intervention was calculated from a healthcare perspective (medical costs), multiplying time logged by the care providers by their hourly salary in Belgium.

The savings of the digital intervention were estimated by assuming that alerts solved digitally prevented medical consultation with a general practitioner, or even readmission.

### 2.3. Statistics

The impact of the intervention was assessed by determining the change between the preoperative and the 6 months timepoints. Analysis of differences in the patient-reported outcomes was performed using an independent samples *t*-test or the Mann–Whitney U test. A significance level of 0.05 was used.

## 3. Results

### 3.1. Participants

A total of 127 patients who were referred to the digital rehabilitation trajectory were analyzed (Figure 1). Fourteen patients did not start the trajectory, and twelve did not continue after surgery. These patients did not use any features of the digital rehabilitation and were thus excluded from further analysis. Fourteen patients dropped out of the digital program for the following reasons: preference for in-person physiotherapy ($n = 11$), unknown ($n = 3$). The system was used for an average of 83 days. Patients' use of the system is shown on the graph in Figure 2. Average adherence with the exercise achievement was 77% over the whole rehabilitation journey. A lower adherence was observed during the first two weeks after surgery (Table 2).

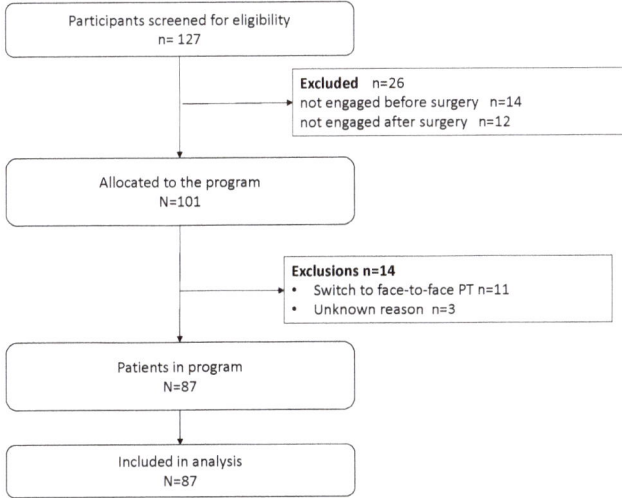

**Figure 1.** Flow diagram.

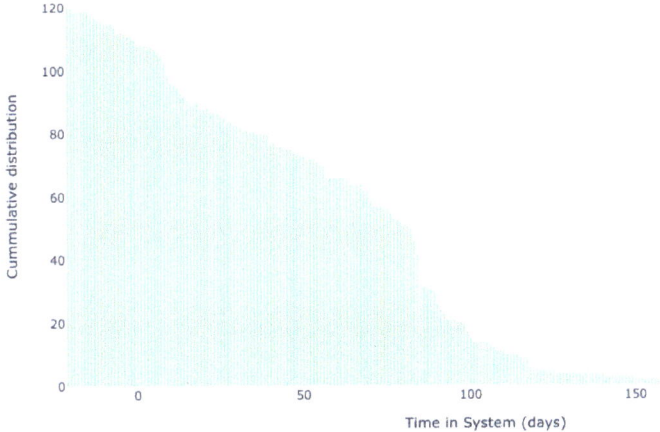

**Figure 2.** Use of digital rehabilitation.

Table 2. Patient engagement over time.

|  | Average | W1-2 | W3-4 | W5-6 | W7-8 | W9-10 | W11-12 |
|---|---|---|---|---|---|---|---|
| Exercises performed (%) | 77 | 67 | 85 | 85 | 77 | 77 | 70 |
| Daily questionnaire filled (%) | 80 | 76 | 89 | 88 | 85 | 82 | 77 |
| Assessment video performed (%) | 71 | 93 | 86 | 75 | 76 | / | / |

W = week post-surgery, /: no standard assessment requested.

### 3.2. Adverse Events

Two patients were readmitted to the hospital for manipulation under anesthesia corresponding to a readmission rate of 2.4%.

A total of 67 alerts were raised through the web-based platforms for 32 patients (39% of the patients). A total of 32 alerts were raised by the patients (48%), and 35 by the physical therapist (52%). The types of alerts are displayed in Figure 3.

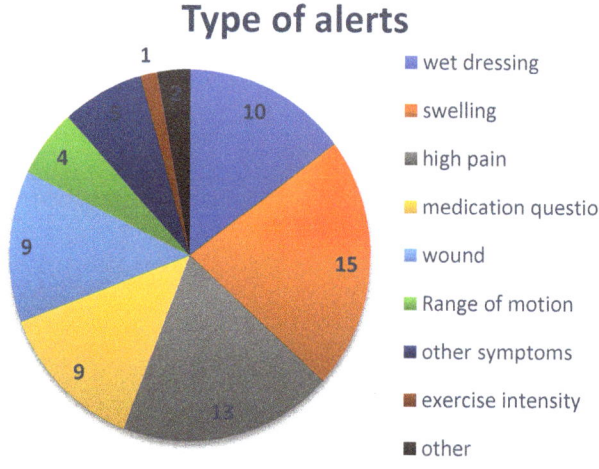

Figure 3. Type of alerts raised by the patient and the physical therapists.

The three most frequent actions were medication change (27%) and wound information and reassurance and referral (15%). The details of doctors actions are displayed in Table 3.. Ten physical consultations were generated by the referrals. Doctor actions through the platform potentially avoided 57 consultations (85% of alerts).

Table 3. Doctor actions in reaction to alerts.

| Category | Frequency n (%) |
|---|---|
| Medication change | 18 (27) |
| Medication info and reassure | 8 (12) |
| Wound care | 6 (9) |
| Wound info and reassure | 10 (15) |
| Symptoms info and reassure | 12 (17) |
| Referral | 10 (15) |
| Other | 3 (4) |

### 3.3. Outcomes

The median active range of motion at 6 weeks post-operation was 105° (SD: 19°).

Significant improvements were seen at 6 months in all KOOS subscales (Table 4), amounting to 14 points in KOOS-Pain, 20 points in KOOS-Symptoms, 22 points in KOOS-Function, and 26 points in KOOS-QoL. The mean QALY gain (measured with the EQ-5D questionnaire) was 0.26 (0.25).

**Table 4.** Patient reported outcomes.

|  | Preop | | 3 Months | | 6 Months | | 6 m/Preop Difference | |
| --- | --- | --- | --- | --- | --- | --- | --- | --- |
|  | Mean | SD | Mean | SD | Mean | SD | Mean | SD |
| Oxford Knee | 24 | 8 | 33 | 8 | 38 | 7 | 14 | 9 |
| KOOS Symptoms | 51 | 18 | 61 | 18 | 70 | 19 | 20 | 21 |
| KOOS Pain | 44 | 19 | 67 | 20 | 78 | 19 | 36 | 20 |
| KOOS ADL | 49 | 20 | 71 | 21 | 78 | 18 | 31 | 22 |
| KOOS QoL | 30 | 18 | 50 | 20 | 56 | 22 | 26 | 27 |
| KSS Satisfaction | 15 | 7 | 25 | 8 | 30 | 8 | 16 | 11 |
| QALY | 0.59 | 0.26 | 0.77 | 0.22 | 0.85 | 0.12 | 0.26 | 0.25 |

SD = Standard deviation, KOOS: Knee Injury and Osteoarthritis Score, ADL: Activities of Daily Living, QoL: Quality of Life, QALY: Quality-Adjusted Life Years.

To the question: "Would you choose digital rehabilitation again?", 89% of the patients answered yes.

### 3.4. Cost–Consequence Analysis

The cost of the digital intervention was EUR 257.5 per person.

This cost comprised the activity tracker (Garmin Vivofit) of EUR 60, an intake cost of EUR 22.5 (15 min by customer support and 15 min by physical therapist), and the average cost of physical therapy follow-up of EUR 170 (average of 18 min per week per patient, standard deviation of 5 min) and medical follow up of EUR 5 (67 interventions of 4 min on average, spread over 86 patients).

Intake costs included onboarding, explanations, and technical support. Intake cost consisted of 15 min remote interactions before surgery with technical support for each participant.

Follow-up costs were calculated from logs that care providers completed during the study. The physical therapists (first-line care provider) logged an average of 18 min per week (SD = 5 min) with each participant (Figure 4). The doctors (second-line care provider) logged 67 instances of solving alerts, with an average of 4 min (SD = 2 min). The time spent by care providers is low because of asynchronous communication, escalation process, and platform efficiency.

The hourly salary in Belgium at the time of the study was 25 EUR/h for technical and customer support, 40 EUR/h for physical therapists, and 100 EUR/h for medical doctors.

The total direct savings of the digital intervention consisted of two aspects: reduced physical therapy costs and reduced unplanned consultations.

Traditional physical therapy after total knee replacement consists of 25 (France) to 41 (Belgium) physical therapy sessions, for an amount of EUR 500 to 1148.

Consultations with a medical doctor cost EUR 27 in Belgium. A total of 57 alerts were digitally solved for 87 patients. This represents a potential amount of EUR 1539 saved, 18 EUR/patient.

Therefore, the total direct saving potential of the digital rehabilitation solution ranges from EUR 252.5 (France) to 900.5 (Belgium).

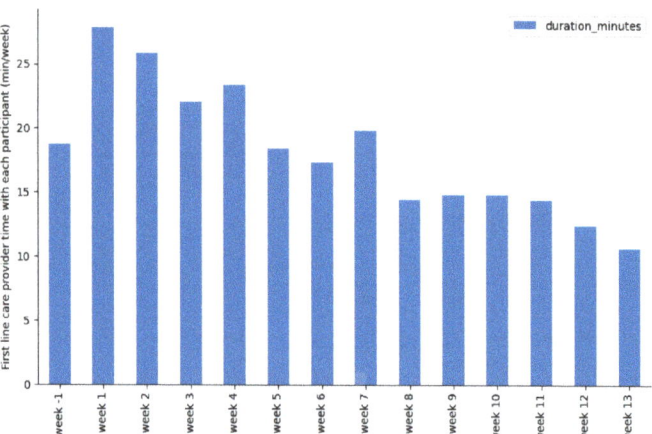

**Figure 4.** First-line care provider time spent with each participant on a weekly basis over the whole rehabilitation period.

## 4. Discussion

The aim of this study was to investigate the engagement, safety, clinical effectiveness, and satisfaction of a personalized and adaptative app-based digital monitoring and rehabilitation program after knee replacement arthroplasty. A high adherence was found, with an average use of 83 days. The complication rate was low, and undesired events were managed remotely in 85% of cases, avoiding unnecessary face-to-face consultations. Clinical scores improved significantly, and most of the patients would choose digital rehabilitation again and recommend it to other patients.

One of the limitations of the study was the absence of a control group (traditional face-to-face rehabilitation program), and the results of this study cannot be compared directly with the results of standard rehabilitation programs. The goal of the study was, however, not to show the superiority or the non-inferiority of this type of program, but to examine the feasibility, the adherence, and the safety regarding the management of the complications and the functional results. Additionally, it was found that 11% of patients stopped the program soon after surgery, mostly due to a lack of physical contact with their physical therapist or because they wanted and needed to preserve a pre-existing relationship with their physical therapist. It is important to highlight the fact that there was no reimbursement difference between the digital care program and a standard in-person physical care program in the study settings (France and Belgium). Therefore, the cost was not a reason to explain the attrition rate, and this outlines the importance of finding ways to reduce it in the future [19].

The attrition rate was low compared to previous studies, reporting between a 7% and 45% attrition rate [12,20]. The results of our study demonstrated a very high adherence level to the proposed exercises (77%). The current literature provides very little evidence surrounding patient adherence to exercise recommendations after TKA, which may also impact the implementation of these interventions [21]. A huge variability exists concerning the type of exercises and the adhesion during the in-person physical therapy programs, except for very-well-designed research studies on the impact of physiotherapy programs after TKA [22]. Therefore, very little data are reported for classic in-person programs during standard clinical practice [5]. Using a mobile application might be ideal to standardize the follow-up of PT interventions after TKA and provide direct quantitative feedback to the patients, which increases their motivation [7]. Usually, exercise adherence decreases over time [16,23], while in our study, it stayed high until the end of the rehabilitation program. It is likely that the closed feedback provided by the data and the human intervention provided to the patients by the physical therapists daily through the app increased their motivation [7,24].

With the global rise in TKA procedures, optimizing postoperative management to enhance patient-reported outcomes is of paramount importance, especially when bundle payment models apply [25]. Shorter hospitalization stays after TKA [26,27] present a need for safer and more personalized postoperative rehabilitation protocols. The most common severe complications which generate important costs are infection, deep vein thrombosis, and manipulation under anesthesia [28,29]. As a result of procedure-related complications, the average 90-day readmission rates vary widely in the literature, ranging from 3.5% to 15.6% in TKA [30,31]. The complication rate in our study was only 2.4% (two readmissions), for manipulations under anesthesia. This low rate might be attributed to the smart alert system that triggered the concerned care provider. In our study, frequent patient concerns regarding wound healing, pain, and medication were frequently observed, requiring attention from the healthcare professionals through the app. Indeed, 39% of the patients expressed concerns, but the ability to seek answers through the mobile application helped to reduce the number of outpatient consultations to only 10. These early referrals through the app with an immediate medical response might have been a factor in preventing more serious complications. These results highlight the potential benefits of implementing digital solutions in healthcare to streamline communication between patients and healthcare professionals, thereby reducing healthcare costs through the reduction of unnecessary consultations while limiting the rate of complications.

The results of our study demonstrated a significant improvement in the Oxford Knee Score, all KOOS sub-scores, and the KSS satisfaction sub-score at 6 months post-surgery. The significant improvements were similar to those previously reported after in-person interventions in Belgium and The Netherlands [32–34], and the population studied was representative of the registry in terms of demographics [35]. The absence of direct comparison with standard protocols in our study limits further conclusions, but the results of our study confirmed previous reports in the literature. In a study by Hardwick-Morris et al., comparing digital rehabilitation to conventional rehabilitation, it was shown that there was no significant difference, after 12 months, in any KOOS or KOOS, JR scores [18]. The study conducted by Timmers et al. demonstrated that the implementation of a digital application post total knee arthroplasty can lead to a significant reduction in daily pain levels and improvement in functional outcomes [20]. Additionally, digital interventions implemented following joint arthroplasty have been found to enhance patient adherence and postoperative satisfaction, making it a potential cornerstone for new pre- and postoperative care pathways in arthroplasty [36]. Based on the results in the literature, it could be said that digital rehabilitation is at least non-inferior to conventional rehab [12].

Introducing new technologies into clinical practice requires careful consideration of patient acceptance and ease of use. In our study, we assessed patient satisfaction with the system and found that the patient promoter/satisfaction score was 89%, indicating a high level of patient acceptance. This finding is consistent with a study by Correia et al., which reported a 90% satisfaction rate [37], or with the study by Scheper et al., which reported high usefulness perceived by patients using an app to specifically monitor wound problems [38]. The convenience of these systems for patients and their caregivers appears to overcome the challenges associated with implementing new technology.

Previous studies have already indicated that digital rehabilitation is an economically viable alternative to traditional in-person care for post knee arthroplasty rehabilitation [39,40]. The biggest difference with previous studies lies in the asynchronous design of the digital rehabilitation used in this study, which reduced the cost drastically. Part of the savings can be used by the healthcare payer to fund the digital platform, so it leads to no costs for the healthcare providers. Furthermore, apart from the cost factor, implementing an asynchronous approach for delivering physical therapy interventions may also alleviate the time constraints imposed on therapists [40], allowing them to dedicate more time to individualizing treatment plans and offering personalized attention to patients with higher needs. More detailed comparison with other studies is difficult, as our follow-up time was relatively limited compared to usual cost studies with a long-term view up to 5 years [14,41]. Indirect costs such as travel costs were not considered. In Belgium, these costs are not covered by insurance. It is likely that the travel reduction participated in the high satisfaction rate of participants.

## 5. Conclusions

In a cohort of patients following a digital rehabilitation program after knee arthroplasty, engagement was high and undesired events were carefully managed through a smart alert system which avoided unnecessary consultations. Clinical improvements were similar to those in other studies, reinforcing the latest review, who stated that digital rehabilitation is non-inferior to conventional rehabilitation. Digital rehabilitation solutions can help to make rehabilitation accessible to everyone and to lower healthcare-related costs by lowering the complication and readmission rate and the rate of unnecessary consultations.

The personalized adaptative human-backed-up app-based digital rehabilitation program for TKA patients presented in this study has a high patient promotor score (satisfaction), as well as a high adherence score (engagement), which make it an ideal rehabilitation partner as it provides good care to the patients (safe and effective) and provides unseen data feedback to the healthcare providers.

**Author Contributions:** Conceptualization, J.L. and S.V.O.; methodology, J.L., A.P., S.P. and S.V.O.; software, A.P.; validation, J.L., A.P., P.A., S.P., P.V.O. and S.V.O.; formal analysis, J.L., A.P. and S.V.O.; investigation, J.L., A.P. and S.V.O.; resources, S.V.O. and P.V.O.; data curation, J.L., A.P., S.V.O. and P.V.O.; writing—original draft preparation, J.L., A.P., P.A., S.P., P.V.O. and S.V.O.; writing—review and editing, J.L., A.P., P.A., S.P., P.V.O. and S.V.O.; visualization, J.L. and A.P.; supervision, S.V.O. and S.P.; project administration, J.L., A.P., S.V.O. and S.P.; funding acquisition, S.V.O. and P.V.O. All authors have read and agreed to the published version of the manuscript.

**Funding:** This research received no external funding.

**Institutional Review Board Statement:** The study was conducted in accordance with the Declaration of Helsinki and approved by the Ethics Committee of Universitair Ziekenhuis Antwerpen (Project ID 5124-27/3/2023).

**Informed Consent Statement:** Informed consent was obtained from all subjects involved in the study.

**Data Availability Statement:** The data presented in this study are available on request from the corresponding author. The data are not publicly available due to privacy reasons.

**Acknowledgments:** The authors acknowledge Cynthia Lapierre and Farah Sinnaeve for their help in the ethics committee application.

**Conflicts of Interest:** P.V.O. is one of the founders of the application studied. J.L. and A.P. are employees of the company commercializing the application. The other authors declare no conflicts of interest.

## References

1. Zhang, W.; Moskowitz, R.W.; Nuki, G.; Abramson, S.; Altman, R.D.; Arden, N.; Bierma-Zeinstra, S.; Brandt, K.D.; Croft, P.; Doherty, M.; et al. OARSI Recommendations for the Management of Hip and Knee Osteoarthritis, Part II: OARSI Evidence-Based, Expert Consensus Guidelines. *Osteoarthr. Cartil.* **2008**, *16*, 137–162. [CrossRef] [PubMed]
2. Kurtz, S.; Ong, K.; Lau, E.; Mowat, F.; Halpern, M. Projections of Primary and Revision Hip and Knee Arthroplasty in the United States from 2005 to 2030. *J. Bone Jt. Surg.* **2007**, *89*, 780–785. [CrossRef]
3. Khan, F.; Ng, L.; Gonzalez, S.; Hale, T.; Turner-Stokes, L. Multidisciplinary Rehabilitation Programmes Following Joint Replacement at the Hip and Knee in Chronic Arthropathy. *Cochrane Database Syst. Rev.* **2008**, *2008*, CD004957. [CrossRef] [PubMed]
4. Marks, R.; Allegrante, J.P. Chronic Osteoarthritis and Adherence to Exercise: A Review of the Literature. *J. Aging Phys. Act.* **2005**, *13*, 434–460. [CrossRef]
5. Bakaa, N.; Chen, L.H.; Carlesso, L.; Richardson, J.; Macedo, L. Reporting of Post-Operative Rehabilitation Interventions for Total Knee Arthroplasty: A Scoping Review. *BMC Musculoskelet. Disord.* **2021**, *22*, 602. [CrossRef]
6. Cyr, M.E.; Etchin, A.G.; Guthrie, B.J.; Benneyan, J.C. Access to Specialty Healthcare in Urban versus Rural US Populations: A Systematic Literature Review. *BMC Health Serv. Res.* **2019**, *19*, 974. [CrossRef]

7. Lang, S.; McLelland, C.; MacDonald, D.; Hamilton, D.F. Do Digital Interventions Increase Adherence to Home Exercise Rehabilitation? A Systematic Review of Randomised Controlled Trials. *Arch. Physiother.* **2022**, *12*, 24. [CrossRef]
8. Schaffer, J.L.; Rasmussen, P.A.; Faiman, M.R. The Emergence of Distance Health Technologies. *J. Arthroplast.* **2018**, *33*, 2345–2351. [CrossRef]
9. Alexandre, D.J.A.; Ramalho, G.S.; Civile, V.T.; Carvas Junior, N.; Cury Fernandes, M.B.; Cacione, D.G.; Trevisani, V.F.M. Telerehabilitation versus Conventional Face-to-Face Land-Based Exercises Following Hip or Knee Arthroplasty (Protocol). *Cochrane Database Syst. Rev.* **2021**. [CrossRef]
10. Correia, F.D.; Nogueira, A.; Magalhães, I.; Guimarães, I.; Moreira, M.; Barradas, I.; Molinos, M.; Teixeira, L.; Tulha, J.; Seabra, R.; et al. Medium-Term Outcomes of Digital Versus Conventional Home-Based Rehabilitation after Total Knee Arthroplasty: Prospective, Parallel-Group Feasibility Study. *JMIR Rehabil. Assist. Technol.* **2019**, *6*, e13111. [CrossRef]
11. Lebleu, J.; Poilvache, H.; Mahaudens, P.; De Ridder, R.; Detrembleur, C. Predicting physical activity recovery after hip and knee arthroplasty? A longitudinal cohort study. *Braz. J. Phys. Ther.* **2021**, *25*, 30–39. [CrossRef] [PubMed]
12. Wang, Q.; Lee, R.L.-T.; Hunter, S.; Chan, S.W.-C. The Effectiveness of Internet-Based Telerehabilitation among Patients after Total Joint Arthroplasty: A Systematic Review and Meta-Analysis of Randomised Controlled Trials. *J. Telemed. Telecare* **2021**, *29*, 247–260. [CrossRef] [PubMed]
13. Kittelson, A.J.; Elings, J.; Colborn, K.; Hoogeboom, T.J.; Christensen, J.C.; van Meeteren, N.L.U.; van Buuren, S.; Stevens-lapsley, J.E. Reference Chart for Knee Flexion Following Total Knee Arthroplasty: A Novel Tool for Monitoring Postoperative Recovery. *BMC Musculoskelet. Disord.* **2020**, *21*, 482. [CrossRef] [PubMed]
14. Konopka, J.F.; Lee, Y.; Su, E.P.; McLawhorn, A.S. Quality-Adjusted Life Years after Hip and Knee Arthroplasty: Health-Related Quality of Life after 12,782 Joint Replacements. *JBJS Open Access* **2018**, *3*, e0007. [CrossRef] [PubMed]
15. Bouckaert, N.; Cleemput, I.; Devriese, S.; Gerkens, S. An EQ-5D-5L Value Set for Belgium. *PharmacoEconomics-Open* **2022**, *6*, 823–836. [CrossRef] [PubMed]
16. Fatoye, F.; Gebrye, T.; Fatoye, C.; Mbada, C. A Systematic Review of Economic Models for Cost Effectiveness of Physiotherapy Interventions Following Total Knee and Hip Replacement. *Physiotherapy* **2022**, *116*, 90–96. [CrossRef]
17. Irina, C.; Mattias, N.; Stefaan, V.D.S.; Nancy, T. *Belgische Richtlijnen Voor Economische Evaluaties en Budget Impact Analyses: Tweede Editie*. Health Technology Assessment (HTA); KCE Reports; Federaal Kenniscentrum voor de Gezondheidszorg (KCE): Brussel, Belgium, 2012; p. 183A. [CrossRef]
18. National Institute for Health and Care Excellence (NICE) Evidence Standards Framework for Digital Health Technologies 2022. Available online: https://www.nice.org.uk/corporate/ecd7 (accessed on 12 May 2023).
19. Eysenbach, G. The Law of Attrition. *J. Med. Internet Res.* **2005**, *7*, e11. [CrossRef]
20. Timmers, T.; Janssen, L.; van der Weegen, W.; Das, D.; Marijnissen, W.-J.; Hannink, G.; van der Zwaard, B.C.; Plat, A.; Thomassen, B.; Swen, J.-W.; et al. The Effect of an App for Day-to-Day Postoperative Care Education on Patients with Total Knee Replacement: Randomized Controlled Trial. *JMIR Mhealth Uhealth* **2019**, *7*, e15323. [CrossRef]
21. Frost, R.; Levati, S.; McClurg, D.; Brady, M.; Williams, B. What Adherence Measures Should Be Used in Trials of Home-Based Rehabilitation Interventions? A Systematic Review of the Validity, Reliability, and Acceptability of Measures. *Arch. Phys. Med. Rehabil.* **2017**, *98*, 1241–1256.e45. [CrossRef]
22. Konnyu, K.J.; Thoma, L.M.; Cao, W.; Aaron, R.K.; Panagiotou, O.A.; Bhuma, M.R.; Adam, G.P.; Balk, E.M.; Pinto, D. Rehabilitation for Total Knee Arthroplasty: A Systematic Review. *Am. J. Phys. Med. Rehabil.* **2023**, *102*, 19–33. [CrossRef]
23. Lewis, M.; Sutton, A. Understanding Exercise Behaviour: Examining the Interaction of Exercise Motivation and Personality in Predicting Exercise Frequency. *J. Sport Behav.* **2011**, *34*, 82–97.
24. Wright, B.J.; Galtieri, N.J.; Fell, M. Non-Adherence to Prescribed Home Rehabilitation Exercises for Musculoskeletal Injuries: The Role of the Patient-Practitioner Relationship. *J. Rehabil. Med.* **2014**, *46*, 153–158. [CrossRef]
25. Nussbaum, S.; McClellan, M.; Metlay, G. Principles for a Framework for Alternative Payment Models. *JAMA* **2018**, *319*, 653–654. [CrossRef] [PubMed]
26. Wainwright, T.W. Enhanced Recovery after Surgery (ERAS) for Hip and Knee Replacement-Why and How It Should Be Implemented Following the COVID-19 Pandemic. *Medicina* **2021**, *57*, 81. [CrossRef] [PubMed]
27. Bradley, B.; Middleton, S.; Davis, N.; Williams, M.; Stocker, M.; Hockings, M.; Isaac, D.L. Discharge on the Day of Surgery Following Unicompartmental Knee Arthroplasty within the United Kingdom NHS. *Bone Jt. J.* **2017**, *99-B*, 788–792. [CrossRef] [PubMed]
28. Healy, W.L.; Della Valle, C.J.; Iorio, R.; Berend, K.R.; Cushner, F.D.; Dalury, D.F.; Lonner, J.H. Complications of Total Knee Arthroplasty: Standardized List and Definitions of The Knee Society. *Clin. Orthop. Relat. Res.* **2013**, *471*, 215–220. [CrossRef]
29. Heo, S.M.; Harris, I.; Naylor, J.; Lewin, A.M. Complications to 6 Months Following Total Hip or Knee Arthroplasty: Observations from an Australian Clinical Outcomes Registry. *BMC Musculoskelet. Disord.* **2020**, *21*, 602. [CrossRef]
30. Jaibaji, M.; Volpin, A.; Haddad, F.S.; Konan, S. Is Outpatient Arthroplasty Safe? A Systematic Review. *J. Arthroplast.* **2020**, *35*, 1941–1949. [CrossRef]
31. Thompson, J.W.; Wignadasan, W.; Ibrahim, M.; Plastow, R.; Beasley, L.; Haddad, F.S. The Introduction of Day-Case Total Knee Arthroplasty in a National Healthcare System: A Review of the Literature and Development of a Hospital Pathway. *Surgeon* **2022**, *20*, 103–114. [CrossRef]

32. Loef, M.; Gademan, M.G.J.; Latijnhouwers, D.A.J.M.; Kroon, H.M.; Kaptijn, H.H.; Marijnissen, W.J.C.M.; Nelissen, R.G.H.H.; Vliet Vlieland, T.P.M.; Kloppenburg, M. Comparison of KOOS Scores of Middle-Aged Patients Undergoing Total Knee Arthroplasty to the General Dutch Population Using KOOS Percentile Curves: The LOAS Study. *J. Arthroplast.* **2021**, *36*, 2779–2787.e4. [CrossRef]
33. LeBrun, D.G.; Martino, B.; Biehl, E.; Fisher, C.M.; Gonzalez Della Valle, A.; Ast, M.P. Telerehabilitation Has Similar Clinical and Patient-Reported Outcomes Compared to Traditional Rehabilitation Following Total Knee Arthroplasty. *Knee Surg. Sport. Traumatol. Arthrosc.* **2022**, *30*, 4098–4103. [CrossRef] [PubMed]
34. Van Onsem, S.; Verstraete, M.; Dhont, S.; Zwaenepoel, B.; Van Der Straeten, C.; Victor, J. Improved Walking Distance and Range of Motion Predict Patient Satisfaction after TKA. *Knee Surg. Sport. Traumatol. Arthrosc.* **2018**, *26*, 3272–3279. [CrossRef] [PubMed]
35. Belgian Hip and Knee Arthroplasty Registry 2015. Available online: https://www.sorbcot.be/attachments/article/5/Rapport%20Orthopride%202017.pdf (accessed on 12 May 2023).
36. Sharareh, B.; Schwarzkopf, R. Effectiveness of Telemedical Applications in Postoperative Follow-Up after Total Joint Arthroplasty. *J. Arthroplast.* **2014**, *29*, 918–922.e1. [CrossRef]
37. Correia, F.D.; Nogueira, A.; Magalhães, I.; Guimarães, J.; Moreira, M.; Barradas, I.; Teixeira, L.; Tulha, J.; Seabra, R.; Lains, J.; et al. Home-Based Rehabilitation with a Novel Digital Biofeedback System versus Conventional In-Person Rehabilitation after Total Knee Replacement: A Feasibility Study. *Sci. Rep.* **2018**, *8*, 11299. [CrossRef]
38. Scheper, H.; Derogee, R.; Mahdad, R.; van der Wal, R.J.P.; Nelissen, R.G.H.H.; Visser, L.G.; de Boer, M.G.J. A Mobile App for Postoperative Wound Care after Arthroplasty: Ease of Use and Perceived Usefulness. *Int. J. Med. Inform.* **2019**, *129*, 75–80. [CrossRef] [PubMed]
39. Fusco, F.; Turchetti, G. Telerehabilitation after Total Knee Replacement in Italy: Cost-Effectiveness and Cost-Utility Analysis of a Mixed Telerehabilitation-Standard Rehabilitation Programme Compared with Usual Care. *BMJ Open* **2016**, *6*, e009964. [CrossRef]
40. Tousignant, M.; Moffet, H.; Nadeau, S.; Mérette, C.; Boissy, P.; Corriveau, H.; Marquis, F.; Cabana, F.; Ranger, P.; Belzile, É.L.; et al. Cost Analysis of In-Home Telerehabilitation for Post-Knee Arthroplasty. *J. Med. Internet Res.* **2015**, *17*, e83. [CrossRef] [PubMed]
41. Serikova-Esengeldina, D.; Glushkova, N.; Abdushukurova, G.; Mussakhanova, A.; Mukhamejanova, A.; Khismetova, Z.; Bokov, D.; Ivankov, A.; Goremykina, M.; Semenova, Y. Cost-Utility Analysis of Total Knee Arthroplasty Alone and in Comparison with Post-Surgical Rehabilitation and Conservative Treatment in the Republic of Kazakhstan. *Cost Eff. Resour. Alloc.* **2022**, *20*, 47. [CrossRef] [PubMed]

**Disclaimer/Publisher's Note:** The statements, opinions and data contained in all publications are solely those of the individual author(s) and contributor(s) and not of MDPI and/or the editor(s). MDPI and/or the editor(s) disclaim responsibility for any injury to people or property resulting from any ideas, methods, instructions or products referred to in the content.

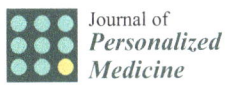

Article

# Cementless Metal-Free Ceramic-Coated Shoulder Resurfacing

James W. Pritchett

Swedish Medical Center, 901 Boren Ave., Suite 711, Seattle, WA 90104, USA; bonerecon@aol.com;
Tel.: +206-779-2590

**Abstract:** Shoulder resurfacing is a versatile, bone-conserving procedure to treat arthritis, avascular necrosis, and rotator cuff arthropathy. Shoulder resurfacing is of interest to young patients who are concerned about implant survivorship and those in need of a high level of physical activity. Using a ceramic surface reduces wear and metal sensitivity to clinically unimportant levels. Between 1989 and 2018, 586 patients received cementless, ceramic-coated shoulder resurfacing implants for arthritis, avascular necrosis, or rotator cuff arthropathy. They were followed for a mean of 11 years and were assessed using the Simple Shoulder Test (SST) and Patient Acceptable Symptom State (PASS). CT scans were used in 51 hemiarthroplasty patients to assess the glenoid cartilage wear. Seventy-five patients had a stemmed or stemless implant in the contralateral extremity. A total of 94% of patients had excellent or good clinical results and 92% achieved PASS. 6% of patients required a revision. A total of 86% of patients preferred their shoulder resurfacing prosthesis over a stemmed or stemless shoulder replacement. The glenoid cartilage wear at a mean of 10 years was 0.6 mm by a CT scan. There were no instances of implant sensitivity. Only one implant was removed due to a deep infection. Shoulder resurfacing is an exacting procedure. It is clinically successful, with excellent long-term survivorship in young and active patients. The ceramic surface has no metal sensitivity, very low wear, and, therefore, it is successful as a hemiarthroplasty.

**Keywords:** shoulder resurfacing; arthroplasty; cementless resurfacing; ceramic-coated implant

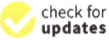

Citation: Pritchett, J.W. Cementless Metal-Free Ceramic-Coated Shoulder Resurfacing. *J. Pers. Med.* **2023**, *13*, 825. https://doi.org/10.3390/jpm13050825

Academic Editor: Johannes Beckmann

Received: 10 April 2023
Revised: 8 May 2023
Accepted: 11 May 2023
Published: 13 May 2023

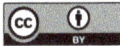

**Copyright:** © 2023 by the author. Licensee MDPI, Basel, Switzerland. This article is an open access article distributed under the terms and conditions of the Creative Commons Attribution (CC BY) license (https://creativecommons.org/licenses/by/4.0/).

## 1. Introduction

The humeral head has been considered a surplus skeletal part and is removed routinely by most surgeons when performing a shoulder implant procedure. Replacement with a metal head attached to a stem placed into the medullary canal of the humerus has been the chosen reconstructive treatment. This may be an unnecessary concession to convention and surgeon's convenience [1–4]. It may not be the best option for every patient. During the initial development of implant procedures, surgeons were concerned about the intrusive nature of the procedures and the amount of metal involved. The biocompatibility of the implant itself was an additional concern. Any implanted material must be durable, capable of excellent functional performance, and biocompatible.

Cup arthroplasty was suggested initially for both the hip and shoulder [5–7]. Resurfacing arthroplasty, or surface replacement, is an evolved technique from cup arthroplasty. In this technique, only the degraded surface of the humeral head is replaced and, when necessary, the glenoid is resurfaced. Although it is easier and less demanding to excise the humeral head and perform a total joint replacement, a resurfacing procedure is more conservative and can be a better option for the patient [8–17].

Humeral head resurfacing is best suited for a young patient with arthritic involvement predominately of the humeral head. It can also be used to treat avascular necrosis and the occasional head-splitting fracture. There are cases in which resurfacing is the best option because there is a deformity or prior surgery with existing hardware in the humerus blocking the placement of a stemmed prosthesis. It can be used in teenagers or in cases with an elevated fear of infection. Contraindications to resurfacing include poor bone quality or unstable soft tissues. The under surface of the implant is coated with a porous surface for ingrowth/ongrowth [8,9,12–15].

In the majority of cases, the humeral resurfacing prosthesis will articulate directly with the preserved glenoid cartilage [8–15]. Therefore, the smoothest possible surface is necessary. Ceramic coating the implant is the best method to achieve this goal (Figure 1).

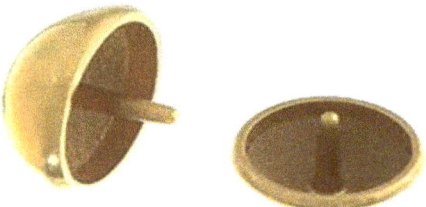

**Figure 1.** Cementless, ceramic-coated shoulder resurfacing implant.

Titanium nitride (TiN) has high hardness and a low friction coefficient. It has been shown to be efficient in reducing the wear of cutting tools. It has been cleared by the Food and Drug Administration as an implant bearing surface and coating (510K 93122). It has much less wear compared to the cobalt chromium implants that are typically used for shoulder replacement and other resurfacing implants. In addition to reduced wear, there are no metal ions released into the tissues and, therefore, no chance of metal sensitivity or an allergic reaction [18–20]. The glenoid component, when needed, is either cemented or porous-backed polyethylene [10,15] (Figure 2).

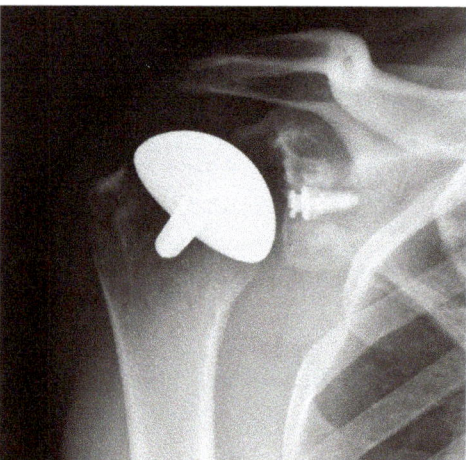

**Figure 2.** AP radiograph of a shoulder resurfacing with a polyethylene glenoid resurfacing component.

This study answered five questions:
- Does cementless, ceramic-coated shoulder resurfacing produce satisfactory function and survivorship?
- What is the wear of ceramic resurfacing prostheses?
- Can a ceramic humeral resurfacing prosthesis produce acceptable outcomes without glenoid resurfacing?
- Do patients prefer shoulder resurfacing to other implant procedures?
- Can a ceramic humeral shoulder resurfacing prosthesis provide acceptable outcomes for rotator cuff arthropathy patients?

## 2. Materials and Methods

The Institutional Review Board approved this retrospective study. The patients reported in this study underwent their shoulder procedures between 1989 and 2018. The patients' function and comfort were assessed using the Simple Shoulder Test (SST) before surgery and at follow-up every other year [4,21]. Patients were followed in person, with video visits, and electronically. We used the SST and the Patient Acceptable Symptom State (PASS) because they allow patients to assess their own function and comfort. The most recent SST score was compared with the preoperative score to assess the outcome. In addition, patients who had a stemmed or stemless prosthesis in their other shoulder were asked which shoulder they preferred. They were also asked the reasons for the preference. Most of our patients were from out of town with an average distance from the clinic of 1160 miles. There were 3 groups of patients:

- Humeral hemiarthroplasty.
- Total resurfacing arthroplasty with a ceramic humeral resurfacing component articulating with a polyethylene glenoid.
- Hemiarthroplasty for rotator cuff arthropathy.

Shared decision-making was used to determine the procedure that a patient preferred. A stem-supported anatomic or reverse total shoulder replacement was performed according to the patient's choice. Additionally, a glenoid component was placed at the time of humeral head resurfacing if there was significant glenoid wear or if this was the patient's choice.

All patients received radiographs. The radiographs were examined to determine component fixation, component position, bone loss, and, if evident, glenoid cartilage wear. A total of 51 hemiarthroplasty patients received CT scans 9–11 years after their surgery to accurately measure the glenoid cartilage wear [22].

Retrieval analysis was performed on implants that were obtained either postmortem or if there was a revision.

### 2.1. The Humeral Head Implant

The titanium alloy $Ti6Al_4V$ humeral implant was straight-stemmed and proportional from 44–56 mm in diameter. Its undersurface was porous-coated with commercially pure titanium plasma spray/beads to give an average pore size of 350 μm and a volume porosity of 30%. The articulating surface was made of titanium alloy coated with a polished 10 μm-thick layer of titanium nitride ceramic (TiN). This polishing was to 0.03 μ before and to 0.04 μ after the TiN coating. The TiN coating was applied using the Physical Vapor Deposition process [18]. When a glenoid component was used, it was Ethylene Oxide sterilized GUR 1020 polyethylene.

### 2.2. Surgical Technique

The resurfacing arthroplasty technique was designed to restore anatomy to the articular surface of the humerus by applying a "cap" over the reamed surface of the humeral head. An anatomic position restored the normal degree of retroversion (average 30°) and valgus (average 140°). This allowed the tuberosities to be maintained with the rotator cuff attachments and a preserved force couple.

When there is rotator cuff tear arthropathy with superior migration of the humeral head but with a still captured humeral head within the coracoacromial arch, resurfacing is possible. An "acetabularized" articulation with the humeral head using both the glenoid and acromion is created. A now smooth surface can allow this articulation with altered mechanics to provide reasonable function while reducing pain. In this situation, the direction of the humeral head reaming may be as high as 170° valgus ("hyper valgus") and a femoral rather than humeral resurfacing device. These are limited goal cases from a functional standpoint. The arm can be raised to eye level.

For both anatomic and rotator cuff arthropathy resurfacing, the operative technique is similar: a deltopectoral approach is used. A limited number of pectoralis fibers can be released to visualize the subscapularis. In cases of cuff tear arthropathy, the upper subscapularis may have eroded; the supraspinatus and infraspinatus are usually retracted medial to the humeral head. The humeral head rides high in the subacromial space but is contained within the subacromial arch. In the more typical cases with an intact or nearly intact rotator cuff, the subscapularis is incised with a stump for later repair. The dissection stops at the rotator cuff interval, avoiding injury to the insertion of the supraspinatus and then the head is dislocated anteriorly. In all cases, great care is taken to preserve the coracoacromial ligament.

Once the humeral head has been delivered into the wound, the well-visualized peripheral osteophytes are removed. A center guide wire is placed at the normal inclination of the humeral head, perpendicular to the apex of the natural articular surface. In cases of cuff tear arthropathy, the guide wire is placed in hyper valgus, which will allow seating over the entire superior humeral surface including the tuberosities. If the biceps are healthy, it is left intact; if not, a tenodesis is performed as part of the closure. The head sizer is placed over the guide wire. Caution should be taken not to start the reamer before full application to the bone to avoid grabbing and fracturing the humeral head or neck. Only the articular surface is reamed down to bleeding bone.

*2.3. Statistical Analysis*

The clinical assessments were based on written responses to the SST [4,21]. These responses were collected through January 2018, preoperatively and postoperatively. The percentage of maximum possible improvements was calculated for the SST score with the following formula: SST total score at the time of follow-up—SST total score preoperatively × 100%/12 points—SST total score preoperatively.

Patients were considered to have achieved a meaningful improvement if the SST increased by at least 30% of the maximum possible improvement. This method avoids the ceiling effect that results from defining minimum clinically important differences. Survivorship was defined as the absence of revision procedures and calculated using a Kaplan–Meier estimator.

The PASS test was used as the more sensitive measure to assess the outcome in this unique and demanding population. The PASS question used was as follows: "Taking in account your shoulder pain and function and how it affects your daily life including your ability to participate in sport and social activities, do you consider your current state acceptable?" PASS determines if a patient improves to the point of getting well.

## 3. Results

The clinical outcomes were reported for three groups of patients:
- Resurfacing hemiarthroplasty.
- Total shoulder resurfacing with a polyethylene glenoid.
- Resurfacing arthroplasty for rotator cuff arthropathy.

*3.1. Shoulder Resurfacing Hemiarthroplasty*

There were 428 patients: 286 (67%) were men, 137 (32%) were women, and 4 (1%) were non-binary. The mean patient age was 52 (standard deviation SD 10.2 years; range, 15–73 years). A total of 158 (37%) had prior surgery on their shoulder. The mean preoperative SST score was 4 (SD 2.5) out of a possible 12 shoulder functions. For the unrevised shoulder followed for a minimum of 5 years (mean 11 years; range 5–30 years), the mean SST score was 10.5 (SD 2.9) of 12 possible positive responses. The median SST was 11 points (interquartile range, 9–12 points). A total of 402 (94%) hemiarthroplasty patients obtained ≥ 30% of the maximum possible improvement in the SST score between the preoperative and peak evaluation. A total of 92% of patients achieved PASS (Table 1). A total of 26 (6%) hemiarthroplasty patients had subsequent procedures: 9 (2%) hemiarthroplasty patients had a revision to add a glenoid component, 5 had revisions to total shoulder replacement, 5 had revisions to a reverse total shoulder replacement, 3 had subscapularis or rotator cuff repairs, 2 had fracture repairs, and 2 had arthroscopic release procedures. There were twenty-three incision infections with three deep infections. There was one dislocation and two fractures. There were five brachial plexopathies and one had a permanent partial median nerve deficit. There was one loose humeral resurfacing implant.

Table 1. Results by procedure type.

| Study Procedure | SST (% Good or Excellent Results) | PASS (% Achieved) | Prosthesis Revision (%) | Complications (n) |
|---|---|---|---|---|
| Resurfacing Hemiarthroplasty | 94 | 92 | 6 | 7 |
| Resurfacing Total Arthroplasty | 90 | 90 | 12 | 3 |
| Stemmed Hemiarthroplasty | 80 | 81 | 15 | 12 |
| Stemmed Total Arthroplasty | 84 | 86 | 12 | 11 |
| Resurfacing Cuff Arthropathy Arthroplasty | 66 | 76 | 6 | 7 |
| Stemmed Reverse Total Shoulder Arthroplasty | 69 | 77 | 11 | 13 |

*3.2. Total Shoulder Resurfacing*

There were 91 patients treated with a total resurfacing shoulder: 51 (56%) were men and 40 (44%) were women. The mean patient age was 64 (SD 10.3 years; range 39–77). A total of 35 (39%) had prior surgery. The mean preoperative SST score was 4 (SD 2.5). For the total shoulder arthroplasty, the mean postoperative SST score was 9.9 (SD 3.1) of 12 possible responses. The median SST was 11 points (interquartile range; 9–12 points). A total of 74 patients (90%) obtained $\geq 30\%$ of the maximum possible improvement in the SST score and 90% achieved PASS (Table 1). A total of nine (12%) total shoulder resurfacing patients had revision procedures: three were to a reverse total shoulder arthroplasty, three were glenoid revisions for loosening (in one instance, the glenoid prosthesis was removed and not replaced), two were rotator cuff repairs, and one was an arthroscopic lysis of adhesions. There were two incision infections and no deep infections. There was one brachial plexopathy that resolved.

*3.3. Rotator Cuff Resurfacing Arthropathy*

For the 67 rotator cuff arthropathy patients, the mean patient age was 67 (SD 10.6 years, range; 51–83 years): 46 (68%) were men, 21 (32%) were women, and 44 (67%) had prior surgery (Figure 3).

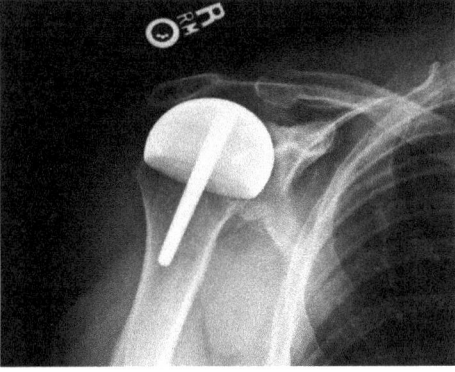

**Figure 3.** This AP shoulder radiograph shows a shoulder resurfacing performed with a full coverage component covering the tuberosities and articulating with the acromion and glenoid.

The mean preoperative SST score for rotator cuff arthropathy was 2.5 (SD 2.5) out of a possible 12. For the rotator cuff arthropathy patients, the mean SST score was 7.7 (SD 4) of 12 possible responses. The median SST was 8 (interquartile range; 5–11 points). A total of 43 (64 %) obtained $\geq$ 30% of the maximum possible improvement in the SST score. A total of 64% achieved PASS. There were three incision infections and one deep infection in a multiply operated shoulder. There were three brachial plexopathies and one had a permanent medial nerve deficit. Of the combined group, 31 patients were lost to follow-up and the outcomes at a minimum of 5 years were reported. Nineteen patients died of causes unrelated to shoulder resurfacing. The number of deaths was less than the actuarial predictions for the general population and were not shared by total shoulder replacement. This was also reported for hip resurfacing [23].

### 3.4. Patient Preference

A total of 55 resurfacing hemiarthroplasty patients had a different prosthesis on the other side: a stemmed total shoulder replacement (19), stemmed hemiarthroplasty (18), total shoulder resurfacing (9), reverse shoulder arthroplasty (7), and resurfacing hemiarthroplasty for rotator cuff arthropathy (2). A total of 11 shoulder arthroplasty patients had a different prosthesis on the other side: stemmed total shoulder replacement (5), stemmed hemiarthroplasty (3), resurfacing hemiarthroplasty (2), and reverse total shoulder arthroplasty (1). A total of 9 rotator cuff arthropathy patients had a different prosthesis on the other side: stemmed total shoulder arthroplasty (3), reverse total shoulder arthroplasty (2), stemmed hemiarthroplasty (2), and resurfacing hemiarthroplasty (2).

A total of 50 out of 55 (90%) of hemiarthroplasty patients preferred their hemiarthroplasty compared to their other shoulder. Three preferred their total resurfacing shoulder or stemmed total shoulder and two had no preference. Eight of the eleven total shoulder resurfacing patients preferred their total shoulder resurfacing to their other shoulder. Two preferred their resurfacing hemiarthroplasty and one had no preference. Six out of nine rotator cuff arthropathy patients preferred their hemiarthroplasty to their other prosthesis, and three preferred their reverse total shoulder arthroplasty (Table 2). The reasons provided were consistent: it feels more natural, it feels more stable, and I can do more with it [24,25]. The operative time for resurfacing hemiarthroplasty was a mean of 24 min longer compared to stemmed hemiarthroplasty. No patient had signs or symptoms of metal sensitivity. Titanium ion concentrations were measured in 39 patients and they were all unmeasurable, indicating low wear and bonding of the ceramic coating.

Table 2. Patient preferences comparison.

| Study Procedure | Study Procedure vs. Prosthesis in Contralateral Shoulder | | |
|---|---|---|---|
| | Prefer Resurfacing | Prefer Stemmed | No Preference |
| Resurfacing Arthroplasty vs. Stemmed Total Arthroplasty | 90% | 5% | 5% |
| Resurfacing Hemiarthroplasty vs. Stemmed Hemiarthroplasty | 70% | 30% | 0% |
| Resurfacing Arthroplasty for Arthropathy vs. Stemmed Total Arthroplasty | 80% | 20% | 10% |

### 3.5. Radiographic Examination

Radiographs showed the humeral resurfacing implant was placed correctly in all cases. There were no implants with loosening or radiolucent lines. There were no areas of osteolysis. The glenohumeral joint space, as visualized on plain films, was maintained. The glenohumeral joint space was measured by a CT scan in 51 hemiarthroplasty patients aged 9–11 years (SD 3 years, range 5–15 years) following surgery. There was a mean decrease of 0.6 mm (range, 0–1.6). There were 12 cases where patients started with < 2 mm of joint space.

*3.6. Retrieval Studies*

A postmortem or revision retrieval analysis was available for nine TiN-coated humeral implants obtained 10 or more years following implantation. The average TiN wear at the head pole of the spherical surface was 1.5 µm, with the remaining 8 µm intact. There were four retrievals of polyethylene glenoid components articulating with TiN humeral components. The maximum polyethylene volumetric wear was 19 mm$^3$/year. There were no areas of polyethylene wear through. There were no instances of reactive synovitis or osteolysis.

## 4. Discussion

Shoulder resurfacing is an effective procedure for increasing function and reducing pain. It has a higher PASS score compared to stemmed supported implants. It is effective both for high-demand patients with an intact rotator cuff as well as for limited-goal patients with rotator cuff arthropathy. Complications from shoulder resurfacing are less frequent and less serious compared to stemmed hemiarthroplasty and stemmed or stemless total shoulder replacement. Only one shoulder resurfacing implant was explanted due to an infection. The other infections were resolved or suppressed with antibiotics. Resurfacing implant survivorship is also better than for stemmed total shoulder replacement. Shoulder resurfacing "burns no bridges". Shoulder resurfacing is a very valuable procedure when the humeral canal is blocked, or when there is an elevated concern for infection.

Revision to stemmed total shoulder replacement or reverse total shoulder replacement was uncommon but uncomplicated and successful when necessary [5,6,8–10,12–17,24]. Shoulder resurfacing is as successful as hemiarthroplasty because glenoid wear is low.

Shoulder resurfacing is a safer and less intrusive procedure compared to total shoulder replacement or hemiarthroplasty with a stemmed or stemless implant. Humeral head resurfacing is also more effective and protective than the "ream and run" procedure. In the "ream and run" procedure, the glenoid is made smooth by reaming but no glenoid implant is placed [4,21,26–28]. A stemmed humeral implant with a prosthetic humeral head articulates with the prepared glenoid. There are three reasons why cementless ceramic shoulder resurfacing is a better solution than "ream and run":

- All the bone is preserved, and the anatomy is restored more precisely. The exact dimension of the humeral head can be recovered, and the retroversion of the shoulder is restored to the anatomic position [29].
- A humeral stem is avoided. Stems create an abnormal load transfer across the shoulder joint with stress shielding of the humerus. Additionally, implantation of a stem increases the difficulties involved if a prosthetic infection occurs. Stemless implants are similar to stemmed implants in that they also produce abnormal forces on the proximal humerus [30,31]. While convenient, stemless implants are not equivalent to head-conserving resurfacing implants.
- A ceramic surface is biocompatible and produces less tissue reaction and wear compared to cobalt chromium. [32]

For patients with rotator cuff arthropathy, shoulder resurfacing offers a less intrusive, lower risk approach than reverse total shoulder replacement. In the event of a reverse total shoulder replacement failing, reconstruction can be very difficult. The results from reverse total shoulder replacement are quite satisfactory and often better than the limited goals of shoulder resurfacing, but the risks are much greater than other shoulder implant procedures [5,27,33].

Patients prefer cementless, ceramic-coated shoulder hemiarthroplasty over total shoulder replacement, reverse total shoulder replacement, and stemmed shoulder hemiarthroplasty. The reasons are a more natural feel and better function. Preference studies are the best way to make comparisons, as all the other variables are controlled [25]. Preference studies have been useful for controlling bias and they have become an accepted method of making comparisons.

It is important to use PASS in assessing the outcome from surgery, as other Patient-Reported Outcome Measures (PROMs) provide some useful information but have their limitations, particularly in highly active individuals. Additionally, survivorship is not the same as a good outcome, and getting better is not equivalent to feeling well. PASS is a more useful method for determining the benefit of a procedure. Achieving PASS may still not reflect a normal state of function. It remains important for both patients and surgeons to recognize that there are limits in our ability to restore shoulder function and measure outcomes. PASS is achieved more often with resurfacing compared to stemmed procedures.

It is very important to use a metal-free implant. A wear simulation test was conducted using 12 specimens to 10 million cycles. The maximum wear patch in the TiN was 1.5 μm compared to the pretest thickness of the coating of 10 μm. The wear penetration, changes to surface roughness, and wear particle analysis showed more than 30 times less wear with ceramic-coated titanium compared to cobalt chromium [34].

Both the retrieval and wear simulator analyses show that a lifetime of use is expected with a ceramic surface. Ceramic wear is much less compared to cobalt chromium. Even without functional or radiographic failure, cobalt chromium wear debris produces synovitis, which can be painful. TiN particles are biocompatible and result in an increase in the proliferation of cells and the affinity of bone to the implant. Cobalt-chromium particles cause osteolysis and chondrolysis. There is lower adhesion of bacteria to TiN surfaces compared to coated or uncoated titanium, cobalt chromium, and polyethylene surfaces and, therefore, a lower infection rate [20,32,33,35,36].

Infections are an important patient concern following any implant arthroplasty procedure. A total of 14.3% of patients raised concerns about incisional infections. Among the patients who were not concerned, the deep prosthetic infection rate was 0.7%. Among patients who had some concerns but no definite superficial infection, the deep infection rate was 3%. For patients with a definite superficial infection, 30% developed a deep prosthetic infection [37]. Infection with resurfacing is less common and much easier to deal with as the medullary space has not been entered. Implant retention is more likely with resurfacing compared to stemmed implant procedures. Only one resurfacing implant was removed for infection, but more than half of the infected stemmed shoulder prostheses were removed.

The results of this study should be reviewed in light of certain limitations. First, all procedures were performed by a surgeon experienced in the technique. Shoulder resurfacing is a demanding technique requiring a close match of the implant to the reshaped native bone. Second, only a single cementless, ceramic-coated implant was used. This implant meets demanding polishing and coating specifications; other implants might not perform as well. Third, most of the patients lived at a distance from the clinic, so we relied on the patients' assessments of their own shoulder functions and comfort using the SST and PASS. Fourth, this procedure was offered to highly motivated patients who understood that their rehabilitation might be long and challenging. Part of the motivation of the patients was the potential to return to a higher level of physical activity. Fifth, there may be patient and surgeon bias in favor of resurfacing due to its bone-conserving nature. Patients are appreciative of the aesthetics of the implant. For the surgeon, however, resurfacing procedures are demanding and take additional time to perform, but since they are hemiarthroplasty procedures, they are compensated at a lower rate compared to total shoulder replacement. For the patient, the expectations are higher, so the outcomes temper the positive bias.

## 5. Conclusions

In conclusion, cementless, ceramic-coated shoulder resurfacing is a valuable procedure. It has conceptual, procedural, functional, wear, and preference advantages over conventional shoulder replacement options in treating advanced articular cartilage damage in the shoulder.

**Funding:** This research received no external funding.

**Institutional Review Board Statement:** The study was conducted in accordance with the Declaration of Helsinki, and approved by the Institutional Review Board of Swedish Medical, Seattle, Washington, USA, S1905-11, 16 November 2011.

**Informed Consent Statement:** Informed consent was obtained from all subjects involved in the study. Written informed consent was obtained from the patient(s) to publish this study.

**Data Availability Statement:** The data generated and analyzed in this study are included in this published article.

**Acknowledgments:** The author acknowledges the editorial assistance of Janet L. Tremaine, ELS, in the preparation of this manuscript.

**Conflicts of Interest:** The author declares no conflict of interest.

# References

1. Gurd, F.B. Surplus parts of the skeleton: A recommendation for the excision of certain portions as a means of shortening the period of disability following trauma. *Am. J. Surg.* **1947**, *74*, 705–720. [CrossRef] [PubMed]
2. Neer, C.S., 2nd. Articular replacement for the humeral head. *J. Bone Jt. Surg. Am.* **1955**, *37*, 215–228. [CrossRef]
3. Neer, C.S., 2nd; Watson, K.C.; Stanton, F.J. Recent experience in total shoulder replacement. *J. Bone Jt. Surg. Am.* **1982**, *64*, 319–337. [CrossRef]
4. Somerson, J.; Matsen, F.A., 3rd. Functional outcomes of the ream-and-run shoulder arthroplasty. A concise follow-up of a previous report. *J. Bone Jt. Surg. Am.* **2017**, *99*, 1999–2003. [CrossRef] [PubMed]
5. Johnson, E.; Egund, N.; Kelly, I.; Rydholm, U.; Lidgren, L. Cup arthroplasty of the rheumatoid shoulder. *Acta Orthop. Scand.* **1986**, *57*, 542–546. [CrossRef] [PubMed]
6. Jónsson, E.; Lidgren, L.; Mjöberg, B.; Rydholm, U.; Selvic, G. Humeral cup fixation in rheumatoid shoulders. Roentgen stereophotogrammetry of 12 cases. *Acta Orthop. Scand.* **1990**, *61*, 116–117. [CrossRef]
7. Scuderi, C. Arthroplasty cup with center pin. *Surg. Gynecol. Obstet.* **1955**, *100*, 631–632.
8. Bailie, D.S.; Llinas, P.J.; Ellenbecker, T.S. Cementless humeral resurfacing arthroplasty in active patients less than fifty-five years of age. *J. Bone Jt. Surg. Am.* **2008**, *90*, 110–117. [CrossRef]
9. Burgess, D.L.; McGrath, M.S.; Bonutti, P.M.; Marker, D.R.; Delanois, R.E.; Mont, M.A. Shoulder resurfacing. *J. Bone Jt. Surg. Am.* **2009**, *91*, 1228–1238. [CrossRef]
10. Copeland, S. The continuing development of shoulder replacement: "reaching the surface". *J Bone Jt. Surg Am* **2006**, *88*, 900–905. [CrossRef]
11. Fuerst, M.; Fink, B.; Rüther, W. The DUROM cup humeral surface replacement in patients with rheumatoid arthritis. *J. Bone Jt. Surg. Am.* **2007**, *89*, 1756–1762. [CrossRef]
12. Rai, P.; Davies, O.; Want, J.; Bigsby, E. Long-term follow-up of the Copeland mark II shoulder resurfacing hemi-arthroplasty. *J. Orthop.* **2015**, *13*, 52–56. [CrossRef] [PubMed]
13. Peebles, L.A.; Arner, J.W.; Haber, D.B.; Provencher, M.T. Glenohumeral resurfacing arthroplasty in young, active patients with end-stage osteoarthritis of the shoulder. *Arthrosc. Tech.* **2020**, *9*, e1315–e1322. [CrossRef]
14. Ibrahim, E.F.; Rashid, A.; Thomas, M. Resurfacing hemiarthroplasty of the shoulder for patients with juvenile idiopathic arthritis. *J. Shoulder Elb. Surg.* **2018**, *27*, 1468–1474. [CrossRef] [PubMed]
15. Pritchett, J.W. Long-Term results and patient satisfaction after shoulder resurfacing. *J Shoulder Elbow Surg.* **2011**, *20*, 771–777. [CrossRef]
16. Rydholm, U.; Sjögren, J. Surface replacement of the humeral head in the rheumatoid shoulder. *J. Shoulder Elbow Surg.* **1993**, *2*, 286–295. [CrossRef]
17. Steffee, A.D.; Moore, R.W. Hemi-resurfacing arthroplasty of the rheumatoid shoulder. *Contemp. Orthop.* **1984**, *9*, 51–59.
18. Pappas, M.J.; Makris, G.; Buechel, F.F. Titanium nitride ceramic film against polyethylene. A 48 million cycle wear test. *Clin. Orthop. Relat. Res.* **1995**, *317*, 64–70.
19. Sovak, G.; Weiss, A.; Gotman, I. Osseointegration of Ti6A1$_4$V alloy implants coated with titanium nitride by a new method. *J. Bone Jt. Surg. Br.* **2000**, *82*, 290–296.
20. Van Raay, J.J.A.M.; Rozing, P.M.; Van Blitterswijk, C.A.; Van Haastert, R.M.; Koerten, H.K. Biocompatibility of wear-resistant coatings in orthopaedic surgery in vitro testing with human fibroblast cell cultures. *J. Mater. Sci. Mater. Med.* **1995**, *6*, 80–84. [CrossRef]
21. Roy, J.S.; Macdermid, J.C.; Faber, K.J.; Drosdowech, D.S.; Athwal, G.S. The simple shoulder test is responsive in assessing change following shoulder arthroplasty. *J. Orthop Sport. Phys. Ther.* **2010**, *40*, 413–421. [CrossRef]
22. Egund, N.; Jonsson, E.; Lidgren, L.; Kelly, I.; Petterson, H. Computed tomography of humeral head cup arthroplasties. A preliminary report. *Acta Radiol.* **1987**, *28*, 71–73. [CrossRef] [PubMed]

23. Kendal, A.R.; Prieto-Alhambra, D.; Arden, N.K.; Carr, A.; Judge, A. Mortality rates at 10 years after metal-on-metal hip resurfacing compared with total hip replacement in England: Retrospective cohort analysis of hospital episode statistics. *BMJ* **2013**, *347*, f6549. [CrossRef] [PubMed]
24. Pritchett, J.W. Inferior subluxation of the humeral head after trauma or surgery. *J. Shoulder Elbow. Surg.* **1997**, *6*, 356–359. [CrossRef] [PubMed]
25. Pritchett, J.W. Hip replacement or hip resurfacing with a highly cross-linked polyethylene acetabular bearing: A qualitative and quantitative preference study. *J. Bone Jt. Surg. Open Access* **2020**, *5*, e0004. [CrossRef] [PubMed]
26. Smith, S.L.; Kennard, E.; Joyce, T.J. Shoulder simulator wear test of five contemporary total shoulder prostheses with three axes of rotation and sliding motion. *Biotribology* **2018**, *13*, 36–41. [CrossRef]
27. Banci, L.; Meoli, A.; Hintner, M.; Bloch, H.R. Wear performance of inverted non-conforming bearings in anatomic total shoulder arthroplasty. *Shoulder Elbow.* **2020**, *12* (Suppl. S1), 40–52. [CrossRef]
28. Gartsman, G.M.; Roddey, T.S.; Hammerman, S.M. Shoulder arthroplasty with or without resurfacing of the glenoid in patients who have osteoarthritis. *J. Bone Jt. Surg. Am.* **2000**, *82*, 26–34. [CrossRef]
29. Hasan, S.S.; Leith, J.M.; Campbell, B.; Kapil, R.; Smith, K.L.; Matsen, F.A., 3rd. Characteristics of unsatisfactory shoulder arthroplasties. *J. Shoulder Elbow Surg.* **2002**, *11*, 431–441. [CrossRef]
30. Pritchett, J.W.; Clark, J.M. Prosthetic replacement for chronic unreduced dislocations of the shoulder. *Clin. Orthop. Relat. Res.* **1987**, *216*, 89–93. [CrossRef]
31. Kumar, S.; Sperling, J.W.; Haidukewych, G.H.; Cofield, R.H. Periprosthetic humeral fractures after shoulder arthroplasty. *J. Bone Joint Surg. Am.* **2004**, *86*, 680–689. [CrossRef] [PubMed]
32. Orr, T.E.; Carter, D.R. Stress analyses of joint arthroplasty in the proximal humerus. *J. Orthop. Res.* **1985**, *3*, 360–371. [CrossRef] [PubMed]
33. Reiner, T.; Bader, N.; Panzram, B.; Bülhoff, M.; Omlor, G.; Kretzer, J.P.; Rais, S.P.; Zeifang, F. In vivo blood metal ion levels in patients after total shoulder arthroplasty. *J. Shoulder Elbow Surg.* **2019**, *28*, 539–546. [CrossRef] [PubMed]
34. Barco, R.; Savvido, O.D.; Sperling, J.W.; Sanchez-Sotelo, J.; Cofield, R.H. Complications in reverse shoulder arthroplasty. *EFORT Open Rev.* **2017**, *13*, 72–80. [CrossRef]
35. Chalmers, P.N.; Rahman, Z.; Romeo, A.A.; Nicholson, G.P. Early dislocation after reverse total shoulder arthroplasty. *J. Shoulder Elbow Surg.* **2014**, *23*, 737–744. [CrossRef]
36. Parsons, I.M., 4th; Millet, P.J.; Warner, J.J. Glenoid wear after shoulder hemiarthroplasty: Quantitative radiographic analysis. *Clin. Orthop. Relat. Res.* **2004**, *421*, 120–125. [CrossRef]
37. Gaine, W.J.; Ramamohan, N.A.; Hussein, N.A.; Hullin, M.G.; McCreath, S.W. Wound infection in hip and knee arthroplasty. *J. Bone Jt. Surg. Br.* **2000**, *82*, 561–565. [CrossRef]

**Disclaimer/Publisher's Note:** The statements, opinions and data contained in all publications are solely those of the individual author(s) and contributor(s) and not of MDPI and/or the editor(s). MDPI and/or the editor(s) disclaim responsibility for any injury to people or property resulting from any ideas, methods, instructions or products referred to in the content.

Article

# Influence of Mechanical Alignment on Functional Knee Phenotypes and Clinical Outcomes in Primary TKA: A 1-Year Prospective Analysis

Dominik Rak *, Lukas Klann, Tizian Heinz, Philip Anderson, Ioannis Stratos, Alexander J. Nedopil and Maximilian Rudert

Orthopädische Klinik König-Ludwig-Haus, Lehrstuhl für Orthopädie der Universität Würzburg, 97074 Würzburg, Germany
* Correspondence: d-rak.klh@uni-wuerzburg.de

**Abstract:** In total knee arthroplasty (TKA), functional knee phenotypes are of interest regarding surgical alignment strategies. Functional knee phenotypes were introduced in 2019 and consist of limb, femoral, and tibial phenotypes. The hypothesis of this study was that mechanically aligned (MA) TKA changes preoperative functional phenotypes, which decreases the 1-year Forgotten Joint (FJS) and Oxford Knee Score (OKS) and increases the 1-year WOMAC. All patients included in this study had end-stage osteoarthritis and were treated with a primary MA TKA, which was supervised by four academic knee arthroplasty specialists. To determine the limb, femoral, and tibial phenotype, a long-leg radiograph (LLR) was imaged preoperatively and two to three days after TKA. FJS, OKS, and WOMAC were obtained 1 year after TKA. Patients were categorized using the change in functional limb, femoral, and tibial phenotype measured on LLR, and the scores were compared between the different categories. A complete dataset of preoperative and postoperative scores and radiographic images could be obtained for 59 patients. 42% of these patients had a change of limb phenotype, 41% a change of femoral phenotype, and 24% a change of tibial phenotype of more than ±1 relative to the preoperative phenotype. Patients with more than ±1 change of limb phenotype had significantly lower median FJS (27 points) and OKS (31 points) and higher WOMAC scores (30 points) relative to the 59-, 41-, and 4-point scores of those with a 0 ± 1 change ($p < 0.0001$ to 0.0048). Patients with a more than ±1 change of femoral phenotype had significantly lower median FJS (28 points) and OKS (32 points) and higher WOMAC scores (24 points) relative to the 69-, 40-, and 8-point scores of those with a 0 ± 1 change ($p < 0.0001$). A change in tibial phenotype had no effect on the FJS, OKS, and WOMAC scores. Surgeons performing MA TKA could consider limiting coronal alignment corrections of the limb and femoral joint line to within one phenotype to reduce the risk of low patient-reported satisfaction and function at 1-year.

**Keywords:** knee arthroplasty; mechanical alignment; clinical outcome; phenotype; level of evidence III; prospective study

## 1. Introduction

Successful TKA has been shown to substantially improve mobility and quality of life in patients with advanced osteoarthritis of the knee. The fact that the procedure of total joint replacement is one of the most successful and effective operations with excellent survivorship of the implants, there are still a considerable percentage of patients with ongoing problems with the replaced joint. Studies reveal that about 15–20% of patients are not satisfied with the implanted knee prosthesis [1,2]. Currently, most of these patients are treated with the mechanical alignment (MA) technique, which is still considered the "gold standard" in knee arthroplasty [3]. In MA, the orientation of the joint line and the bone resections are usually not evaluated and measured, as the resection thickness does not influence surgical decision making. However, one reason for the discomfort of a considerable proportion of the patients might be the change in the native orientation of the joint line and, consequently, a change in ligament balancing. To better evaluate the joint line and to understand how far this might influence the outcome, a lot of research and analysis was done, and the concept of phenotypes was established. This classification confirms a wide variability between individuals and challenges the standard of MA [4–6].

Functional phenotypes of the limb, femur, and tibia have been introduced by Hirschmann et al. to provide a contemporary classification of normal coronal limb and knee alignment [7,8]. Functional phenotypes categorize the hip-knee-ankle (HKA) angle, femoral mechanical angle (FMA), and tibial mechanical angle (TMA) within intervals of 3°. One remarkable finding of their work was that only 5.6% of non-osteoarthritic males and 3.6% of non-osteoarthritic females exhibit limb and knee alignment characteristics targeted by mechanically aligned (MA) total knee arthroplasty (TKA) [8].

MA sets the femoral component perpendicular to the femoral mechanical axis, which changes the pre-arthritic distal femoral joint line of most patients because the orientation of this line varies from −6° varus to 6° valgus relative to the femoral mechanical axis in the non-osteoarthritic knee [7,9–12]. When performing MA TKA in 84% of patients that have a pre-arthritic neutral or valgus femoral phenotype (FMA > 91.5°), the femoral phenotype will change by at least one category [7]. In addition, MA sets the tibial component perpendicular to the tibial mechanical axis, which changes the pre-arthritic tibial joint line in most patients because the orientation of this line varies from −9° varus to 3° valgus relative to the tibial mechanical axis in the non-osteoarthritic knee [7,13]. When performing MA TKA in 71% of patients with a pre-arthritic tibial joint orientation different from perpendicular to the tibial mechanical axis, the tibial phenotype will change at least one category [7].

The limb, femoral, and tibial phenotypes in osteoarthritic knees are differently distributed than in healthy non-arthritic knees, with higher deviations from neutral phenotypes [14]. Consequently, it can be expected that any alignment strategy in TKA will change most patients' osteoarthritic limb, femoral, and tibial phenotype regardless of whether the target of the alignment strategy is to restore the patient's pre-arthritic alignment, i.e., kinematic alignment (KA), or to create perpendicular joint lines in relation to the corresponding mechanical axis, i.e., MA [15].

Recently, a study concluded that the MA-induced change of the patient's joint line obliquity and arithmetic HKA angle did not influence patient outcome [16]. This study used an alignment classification system termed coronal alignment of the knee (CPAK), which groups joint line obliquity and the arithmetic HKA angle (an angle computed from the femoral and tibial joint line orientation in relation to the mechanical axis of the corresponding bone) in nine phenotypes [17]. Because joint line obliquity is categorized (e.g., apex distal, neutral, apex proximal) and the arithmetic HKA angle is categorized (e.g., varus, neutral, valgus), it is not sensitive to changes within one category. In contrast, the classification system of functional limb, femoral, and tibial phenotypes is quantitative and, therefore, could help identify the magnitude of phenotype category change that lowers clinical outcome scores.

Assessing whether a change of functional phenotype adversely affects clinical outcomes requires knowing the minimum clinically important difference (MCID) difference of patient-reported questionnaires. The MCID is the smallest change in score that patients perceive as meaningful, which would cause clinicians to consider modifications in their treatment approach. For example, representative MCID values are 13 points for the Forgotten Joint Score (FJS), 3–5 points for the Oxford Knee Score (OKS), and 10 points for the Western Ontario and McMaster Universities Osteoarthritis Index (WOMAC) score [18–20].

A literature review found no reports of MA TKA that assessed the change in functional phenotype and whether the change adversely affected clinical outcome scores. Accordingly, this prospective study determined the proportion of patients with a change of functional limb, femoral, and tibial phenotype after MA TKA and which change caused a low 1-year

Forgotten Joint (FJS) and Oxford Knee (OKS) and high WOMAC score. A follow-up period of one year seemed reasonable because knee function reaches a plateau within the first postoperative year and remains stable in the following years [21–24].

## 2. Materials and Methods

An institutional review board approved this prospective study (IRB-189/19). The lead author (DR) enlisted four experienced academic knee arthroplasty specialists who each supervised a cemented primary MA TKA on 20 consecutive patients with end-stage osteoarthritis using conventional manual instrumentation and a posterior cruciate ligament retaining implant design (Triathlon Stryker, Kalamazoo, MI, USA). Excluded were patients with avascular necrosis, septic arthritis, prior intra-articular fracture, or a severe preoperative knee deformity that required revision components to restore stability. Patients with no pre-operative or postoperative long-leg radiographs (LLR) were also excluded. In addition, surgeons recorded pre-operative values of body mass index (BMI), knee extension, knee flexion, Oxford Knee Score (OKS), and Western Ontario and McMaster Universities Arthritis Index (WOMAC) (100 worst, 0 best) on each patient.

The following describes the key points of the surgical technique. After exposing the knee, the surgeon classified the primary location of the osteoarthritic as medial (i.e., varus deformity), lateral (i.e., valgus deformity), or patellofemoral. The distal femoral resection guide, set at $6°$ of valgus relative to a rod inserted into the intramedullary canal, was seated flush with the most distal condyle of the femur, which determined the varus-valgus (V-V) joint line orientation of the femoral component. The saw slot of an extramedullary tibial resection guide set perpendicular to the mechanical axis of the tibia was positioned 8 mm distal to intact cartilage on the tibial articular surface, which determined the V-V joint line orientation of the tibial component. The surgeon, at their discretion, resurfaced the patella and released ligaments to balance the TKA.

On LLR obtained before and three days after MA TKA, the following angles were computed on the operated limb: (1) The HKA angle measured between the lines connecting the centers of the femoral head, the knee, and the talus, (2) the FMA measured between the femoral mechanical axis and a tangent to the distal femoral condyles, (3) the TMA measured between the tibial mechanical axis and a tangent to the proximal tibia joint surface or the tibial baseplate. Each angle was assigned to a phenotype category [7,8,14].

One year postoperatively, the surgeon sent the FJS, OKS, and WOMAC questionnaires to each patient. Those that filled out each questionnaire were included in this study.

*Statistical Analysis*

The Shapiro-Wilk test determined the normality of the dependent variables. The mean ± standard deviation (SD) and median and interquartile range (IQR) described normal and non-normal dependent variables (JMP Pro, 16.2.0, www.jmp.com, accessed on 23 February 2023). Based on pre- and postoperative HKA angle, FMA, and TMA measurements, patients were assigned to a pre- and postoperative phenotype category, and the change in phenotype category was computed. For each phenotype, the Wilcoxon/Kruskal–Wallis test determined the significance of the difference in the one-year FJS, OKS, and WOMAC scores between each change in the phenotype category. Significance was set at $p < 0.05$.

## 3. Results

Of the 83 eligible patients, 11 patients did not receive a postoperative LLR. Thirteen patients did not return the one-year clinical outcome questionnaires, leaving 59 patients for final data analysis. Table 1 shows the years each surgeon practiced TKA and the preoperative patient characteristics and function scores for those patients treated by each surgeon. There were no significant differences in the proportion of females to males, mean age, mean BMI, the proportion of varus, valgus, and patellofemoral deformities, and preoperative OKS and WOMAC scores between surgeons. Table 2 shows the one-year median FJS, OKS, and WOMAC scores were not significantly different between the patients treated by each surgeon. Hence, this study combined the patients for analysis.

**Table 1.** Pre-operative patient characteristics and function scores for the patients treated by each surgeon.

|  | Surgeon 1 | Surgeon 2 | Surgeon 3 | Surgeon 4 | p-Value |
|---|---|---|---|---|---|
| Years of Practice | 30 | 22 | 17 | 14 | |
|  | Patients' Preoperative Characteristics and Function Scores | | | | |
|  | Number of Patients (N) | | | | |
| Female/Male | 6/10 | 8/7 | 8/7 | 7/6 | $p = 0.7520$ ** |
| Preoperative Deformity: Varus/Valgus/Patellofemoral | 12/4/0 | 12/2/1 | 13/2/0 | 11/2/0 | $p = 0.8108$ ** |
|  | Mean ± Standard Deviation | | | | |
| Age (years) | 67 ± 9 | 68 ± 7 | 63 ± 7 | 66 ± 13 | $p = 0.5266$ * |
| BMI [1] | 29 ± 8 | 33 ± 6 | 31 ± 5 | 33 ± 8 | $p = 0.3121$ * |
| Knee Extension (deg) | 3 ± 4 | 4 ± 6 | 2 ± 3 | 3 ± 4 | $p = 0.6768$ * |
| Knee Flexion (deg) | 112 ± 10 | 111 ± 8 | 104 ± 11 | 105 ± 10 | $p = 0.0597$ * |
| Oxford Knee Score (48 best, 0 worst) | 21 ± 4 | 20 ± 5 | 19 ± 5 | 23 ± 6 | $p = 0.1875$ * |
| WOMAC [2] (0 best, 96 worst) | 43 ± 14 | 48 ± 12 | 49 ± 18 | 45 ± 19 | $p = 0.5935$ * |

[1] Body-Mass-Index; [2] Western Ontario and McMaster Universities Arthritis Index; * ANOVA determined differences between surgeons; ** Pearson's Chi-Square Test determined differences between surgeons.

**Table 2.** Postoperative patient function scores for the patients treated by each surgeon.

|  | Surgeon 1 | Surgeon 2 | Surgeon 3 | Surgeon 4 | p-Value |
|---|---|---|---|---|---|
| Number of patients (N) with 1-year follow-up | 16 | 15 | 15 | 13 | |
|  | Median and [IQR] [1] of Postoperative Function Scores | | | | |
| Forgotten Joint Score (100 best, 0 worst) | 45 [31 to 73] | 60 [15 to 69] | 33 [25 to 77] | 44 [28 to 89] | $p = 0.4692$ * |
| Oxford Knee Score (48 best, 0 worst) | 35 [31 to 45] | 37 [27 to 41] | 40 [27 to 45] | 36 [31 to 43] | $p = 0.3257$ * |
| WOMAC [2] (0 best, 96 worst) | 13 [6 to 16] | 17 [9 to 41] | 11 [4 to 22] | 13 [4 to 28] | $p = 0.8263$ * |

[1] Interquartile Range [IQR] [2] Western Ontario and McMaster Universities Arthritis Index; * Kruskal-Wallis Test determined differences between surgeons.

The pre- and postoperative functional phenotype distribution is illustrated in Figure 1. Remarkably, 42% of the HKA phenotype and 41% of the FMA phenotype, but only 25% of the TMA phenotype were changed to more than one category by MA TKA (Figure 1).

For the one-year FJS, patients with a HKA phenotype change of more than one category had a significantly lower median score of 27 points relative to the 59-point score of those with no or only one category change ($p = 0.0002$) (Figure 2). In addition, patients with a FMA phenotype change of more than one category had a significantly lower median score of 28 points relative to the 69-point score of those with no or only one category change ($p < 0.0001$). A change in TMA phenotype had no effect on the FJS.

For the one-year OKS, patients with a HKA phenotype change of more than one category had a significantly lower median score of 31 relative to the 41-point score of those with a no or only one category change ($p < 0.0001$) (Figure 3). In addition, patients with a FMA phenotype change of more than one category had a significantly lower median score of 32 points relative to the 40-point score of those with no or only one category change ($p < 0.0001$). A change in TMA phenotype had no effect on the OKS.

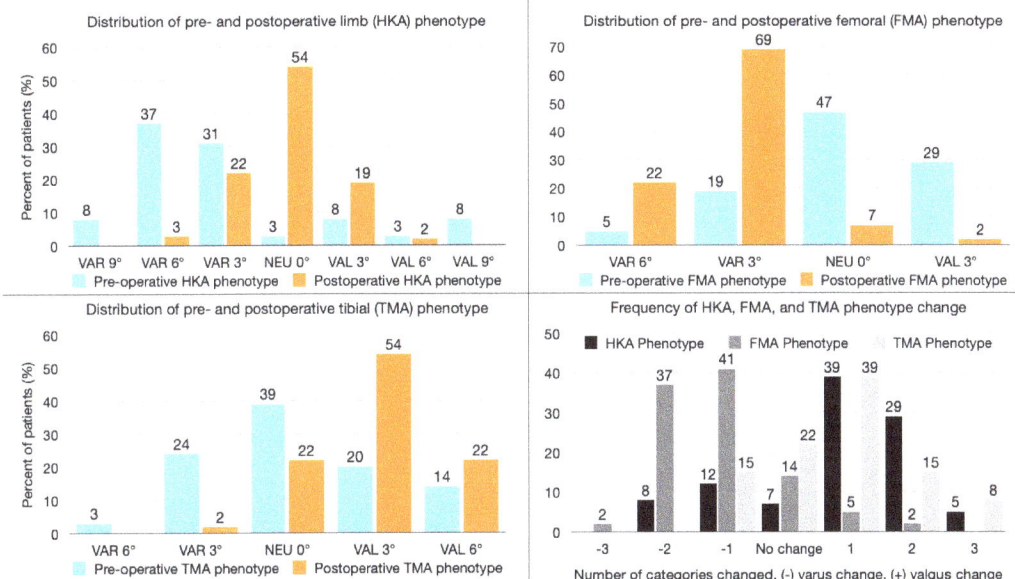

**Figure 1.** The composite shows the distribution of limb (**top left graph**), femoral (**top right graph**), and tibial (**bottom left graph**) phenotypes before and after mechanically aligned total knee arthroplasty (MA TKA). The number of categories MA TKA changed in each functional phenotype is depicted in the (**bottom right graph**).

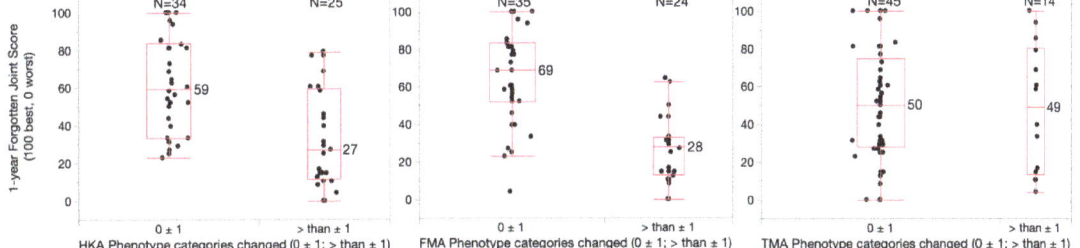

**Figure 2.** Boxplots show the Forgotten Joint Score (FJS) (100 best, 0 worst) of patients who had a phenotype change of fewer than two categories and of more than one category. The median FJS of patients with more than 1 category change of the limb (HKA) and femoral (FMA) phenotype was significantly lower by at least 2 times the 13-point MCID relative to patients whose phenotype changed only one category or less ($p = 0.0002$ (HKA) and $<0.0001$ (FMA)). A change of the tibial (TMA) phenotype of more than one category was less frequent and did not lower the FJS.

For the one-year WOMAC, patients with a HKA phenotype change of more than one category had a significantly higher median score of 30 points relative to the 10-point score of those with no or only one category change ($p = 0.0002$) (Figure 4). In addition, patients with a FMA phenotype change of more than one category had a significantly higher median score of 24 points relative to the 8-point score of those with no or only one category change ($p < 0.0001$). A change in TMA phenotype had no effect on the WOMAC score.

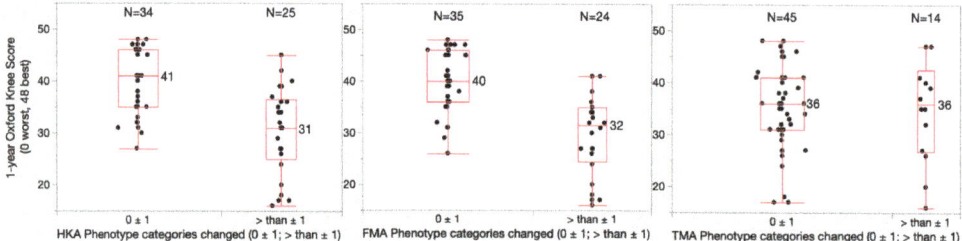

**Figure 3.** Boxplots show the Oxford Knee Score (OKS) (48 best, 0 worst) of patients who had a phenotype change of fewer than two categories and of more than one category. The median OKS of patients with more than 1 category change of the limb (HKA) and femoral (FMA) phenotype was significantly lower by at least once the 5-point MCID relative to patients whose phenotype changed only one category or less ($p < 0.0001$). A change of the tibial (TMA) phenotype of more than one category was less frequent and did not lower the OKS.

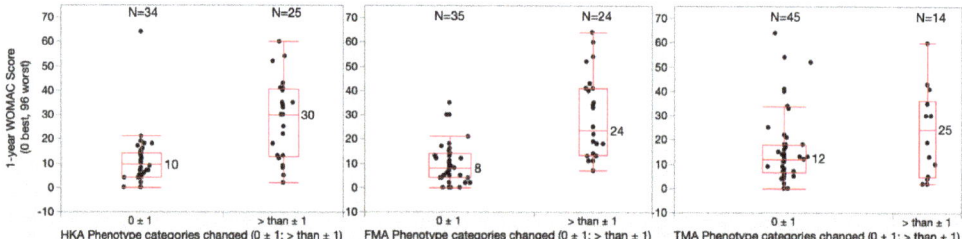

**Figure 4.** Boxplots show the WOMAC score (0 best, 96 worst) of patients who had a phenotype change of fewer than two categories and of more than one category. The median WOMAC score of patients with more than 1 category change of the limb (HKA) and femoral (FMA) phenotype was significantly higher by at least once the 10-point MCID relative to patients whose phenotype changed only one category or less ($p = 0.0002$ (HKA) and <0.0001 (FMA)). A change of the tibial (TMA) phenotype of more than one category was less frequent and did not increase the WOMAC score.

To better analyze whether other factors or variables influence the postoperative outcome after total knee arthroplasty, we added a simple regression analysis that showed that only age, BMI, Preoperative OKS, and preoperative FMA influenced the postoperative outcome, which is already well-known in literature [25–27]. In addition, we performed a Student *t*-test to analyze if these variables have an influence or difference in the two groups displaying the change in phenotype categories. As displayed in Table 3 it showed that none of the variables that influence postoperative outcomes in general have a significant difference in the two groups, whether in the HKA, FMA, or TMA phenotype change group.

**Table 3.** Analysis of the distribution of independent variables that influence postoperative outcomes with respect to the two Phenotype change groups.

|  | HKA Phenotype Categories Change $0 \pm 1$ | HKA Phenotype Categories Change More Than $\pm 1$ | *p*-Value |
|---|---|---|---|
|  | Mean ± Standard Deviation | | |
| Age | 67.2 ± 8.9 | 64.7 ± 9.1 | $p = 0.2927$ * |
| BMI | 31.7 ± 7.4 | 31.6 ± 6.0 | $p = 0.9712$ * |
| Preop Oxford | 21.2 ± 4.2 | 19.8 ± 5.7 | $p = 0.3138$ * |
| Preop FMA | 92.7 ± 2.0 | 92.6 ± 2.6 | $p = 0.9387$ * |

\* *t*-Test determined differences between the two groups who had a phenotype change of fewer than two categories and of more than one category.

## 4. Discussion

The most important findings of the present study were that changing the patient's functional limb and femoral phenotype by more than one category significantly lowered clinical outcome scores, while changing the patient's functional tibial phenotype has a negligible effect on clinical outcome scores.

To the authors' knowledge, this is the first study evaluating the impact of changing the patient's functional limb and knee phenotype on clinical outcomes after MA TKA. This study confirms that a too vigorous change in a patient's limb and knee alignment reflects poorly on clinical outcome [15,28–30]. The changes of the phenotype and, in that sense, a change of the joint line and, thereby, a change of the soft tissue tension may have a distinct impact on the short and long-term outcome. The change in soft tissue balancing is one key point in the discussion of different alignment strategies for knee arthroplasty. A different pressure distribution, soft tissue change, and change of joint alignment might lead to ligament imbalance which might be one reason for dissatisfaction after TKA [31–33].

To address that concern, multiple alternative alignment techniques have evolved, including unrestricted KA, which aims to restore the patient's pre-arthritic alignment without limitations, and functional alignment, which aims to restore the pre-arthritic alignment within defined boundaries, while minimizing changes to the joint line orientation and soft tissue releases [34,35].

While the present study compared pre- and postoperative functional phenotypes (i.e., alignment), it did not evaluate how MA TKA changed patients' pre-arthritic functional phenotypes. Osteoarthritis changes functional phenotype distribution with a wider deviation from neutral [14]. The patient's pre-operative limb, femoral, and tibial phenotype is, therefore, not an adequate target when planning a TKA. However, the results from the present study indicate that patient-reported outcome scores are sensitive to a change of limb and femoral phenotype beyond one category, which could help surgeons performing functional alignment to further personalize their alignment boundaries by avoiding phenotype changes of more than one category [29].

An unexpected result from the present study is that a change in the tibial phenotype did not alter clinical outcome scores. This finding indicates that postoperative patient function is more sensitive to the restoration of pre-arthritic limb alignment and femoral joint line orientation, which corresponds to the concept of unrestricted KA [36]. A principle of unrestricted KA is to restore the flexion–extension (FE) axis of the tibia, which is located within the femoral condyles [9,37].

The present study can help understand why using robotic assistance in MA TKA does not improve patient-reported function beyond the threshold of MCID [38–40]. While robotic assistance or patient-specific instrumentation (PSI) improves the accuracy of component positioning to the MA TKA target, it does not necessarily result in substantial advantages concerning patient functionality [41–43]. Executing MA TKA with high accuracy consistently changes functional phenotypes in more than one category and consequently exposes the patient to an increased risk of inferior clinical outcomes.

The present study has several limitations. First, only one implant system was used to treat the patients in the present study. To generalize the results from this study, surgeons performing MA TKA with other implant systems could measure functional phenotypes and assess whether a change in functional phenotype beyond one category causes a drop in patient-reported outcome scores one year after TKA. Finally, the frequency and extent of soft tissue releases were not included in the data analysis of this study. Because alternative alignment techniques strive to reduce the frequency and extent of soft tissue releases during TKA, it might be of interest whether the change in functional phenotypes is associated with the frequency and extent of soft tissue releases and whether the soft tissue release itself influences patient-reported outcomes. Future studies shall answer this question.

## 5. Conclusions

When performing MA TKA, surgeons should recognize the adverse consequences of changing the patient's presurgical limb and femoral phenotype by two or more categories, as this significantly lowered patient-reported outcomes after one year. If surgeons use robotic instrumentation or navigation to align a TKA, it would be worth considering setting alignment targets that avoid a phenotype change of more than one category.

**Author Contributions:** Conceptualization, D.R., A.J.N. and M.R.; methodology, D.R., A.J.N. and M.R.; software, A.J.N.; validation, D.R., A.J.N. and M.R.; formal analysis, A.J.N.; investigation, D.R., L.K., T.H., P.A., I.S. and A.J.N.; data curation, D.R., L.K., A.J.N. and M.R.; writing—original draft preparation, D.R. and A.J.N.; writing—review and editing, D.R., A.J.N., I.S. and M.R.; visualization, D.R., L.K., I.S. and A.J.N.; supervision, M.R. All authors have read and agreed to the published version of the manuscript.

**Funding:** This research received no external funding.

**Institutional Review Board Statement:** This study was conducted in accordance with the Declaration of Helsinki and approved by the German Institutional Review Board (Ethik-Kommission der Universität Würzburg, Number: 20220720 01, 24 November 2022).

**Informed Consent Statement:** Informed consent was obtained from all subjects involved in this study.

**Data Availability Statement:** The data sets to support the findings of this study are included within the article, including figures and tables. Any other data used to support the findings of this study are available from the corresponding authors upon request.

**Conflicts of Interest:** The authors declare no conflict of interest.

## References

1. Bourne, R.B.; Chesworth, B.M.; Davis, A.M.; Mahomed, N.N.; Charron, K.D. Patient satisfaction after total knee arthroplasty: Who is satisfied and who is not? *Clin. Orthop. Relat. Res.* **2010**, *468*, 57–63. [CrossRef] [PubMed]
2. Noble, P.C.; Conditt, M.A.; Cook, K.F.; Mathis, K.B. The John Insall Award: Patient expectations affect satisfaction with total knee arthroplasty. *Clin. Orthop. Relat. Res.* **2006**, *452*, 35–43. [CrossRef] [PubMed]
3. Roussot, M.A.; Vles, G.F.; Oussedik, S. Clinical outcomes of kinematic alignment versus mechanical alignment in total knee arthroplasty: A systematic review. *EFORT Open Rev.* **2020**, *5*, 486–497. [CrossRef]
4. Hirschmann, M.T.; Hess, S.; Behrend, H.; Amsler, F.; Leclercq, V.; Moser, L.B. Phenotyping of hip-knee-ankle angle in young non-osteoarthritic knees provides better understanding of native alignment variability. *Knee Surg. Sports Traumatol. Arthrosc.* **2019**, *27*, 1378–1384. [CrossRef] [PubMed]
5. MacDessi, S.J.; Griffiths-Jones, W.; Chen, D.B.; Griffiths-Jones, S.; Wood, J.A.; Diwan, A.D.; Harris, I.A. Restoring the constitutional alignment with a restrictive kinematic protocol improves quantitative soft-tissue balance in total knee arthroplasty: A randomized controlled trial. *Bone Jt. J.* **2020**, *102*, 117–124. [CrossRef] [PubMed]
6. Pagan, C.A.; Karasavvidis, T.; Lebrun, D.G.; Jang, S.J.; MacDessi, S.J.; Vigdorchik, J. Geographic Variation in Knee Phenotypes Based on the Coronal Plane Alignment of the Knee (CPAK) Classification: A Systematic Review. *J. Arthroplast.* **2023**, in press. [CrossRef]
7. Hirschmann, M.T.; Moser, L.B.; Amsler, F.; Behrend, H.; Leclercq, V.; Hess, S. Phenotyping the knee in young non-osteoarthritic knees shows a wide distribution of femoral and tibial coronal alignment. *Knee Surg. Sports Traumatol. Arthrosc.* **2019**, *27*, 1385–1393. [CrossRef]
8. Hirschmann, M.T.; Moser, L.B.; Amsler, F.; Behrend, H.; Leclerq, V.; Hess, S. Functional knee phenotypes: A novel classification for phenotyping the coronal lower limb alignment based on the native alignment in young non-osteoarthritic patients. *Knee Surg. Sports Traumatol. Arthrosc.* **2019**, *27*, 1394–1402. [CrossRef]
9. Eckhoff, D.G.; Bach, J.M.; Spitzer, V.M.; Reinig, K.D.; Bagur, M.M.; Baldini, T.H.; Flannery, N.M. Three-dimensional mechanics, kinematics, and morphology of the knee viewed in virtual reality. *J. Bone Jt. Surg. Am.* **2005**, *87* (Suppl. S2), 71–80.
10. Gu, Y.; Howell, S.M.; Hull, M.L. Simulation of total knee arthroplasty in 5 degrees or 7 degrees valgus: A study of gap imbalances and changes in limb and knee alignments from native. *J. Orthop. Res.* **2017**, *35*, 2031–2039. [CrossRef]
11. Niki, Y.; Sassa, T.; Nagai, K.; Harato, K.; Kobayashi, S.; Yamashita, T. Mechanically aligned total knee arthroplasty carries a risk of bony gap changes and flexion-extension axis displacement. *Knee Surg. Sports Traumatol. Arthrosc.* **2017**, *25*, 3452–3458. [CrossRef] [PubMed]
12. Singh, A.K.; Nedopil, A.J.; Howell, S.M.; Hull, M.L. Does alignment of the limb and tibial width determine relative narrowing between compartments when planning mechanically aligned TKA? *Arch. Orthop. Trauma Surg.* **2018**, *138*, 91–97. [CrossRef] [PubMed]

13. Hashemi, J.; Chandrashekar, N.; Gill, B.; Beynnon, B.D.; Slauterbeck, J.R.; Schutt, R.C., Jr.; Mansouri, H.; Dabezies, E. The geometry of the tibial plateau and its influence on the biomechanics of the tibiofemoral joint. *J. Bone Jt. Surg. Am.* **2008**, *90*, 2724–2734. [CrossRef] [PubMed]
14. Jenny, J.Y.; Baldairon, F.; Hirschmann, M.T. Functional knee phenotypes of OA patients undergoing total knee arthroplasty are significantly more varus or valgus than in a non-OA control group. *Knee Surg. Sports Traumatol. Arthrosc.* **2022**, *30*, 2609–2616. [CrossRef]
15. Karasavvidis, T.; Pagan, C.; Haddad, F.; Hirschmann, M.; Pagnano, M.; Vigdorchik, J. Current Concepts in Alignment in Total Knee Arthroplasty. *J. Arthroplast.* **2023**, in press. [CrossRef] [PubMed]
16. Sappey-Marinier, E.; Batailler, C.; Swan, J.; Schmidt, A.; Cheze, L.; MacDessi, S.J.; Servien, E.; Lustig, S. Mechanical alignment for primary TKA may change both knee phenotype and joint line obliquity without influencing clinical outcomes: A study comparing restored and unrestored joint line obliquity. *Knee Surg Sports Traumatol. Arthrosc.* **2022**, *30*, 2806–2814. [CrossRef]
17. MacDessi, S.J.; Griffiths-Jones, W.; Harris, I.A.; Bellemans, J.; Chen, D.B. Coronal plane alignment of the knee (CPAK) classification: A new system for describing knee phenotypes. *Bone Jt. J.* **2021**, *103*, 329–337. [CrossRef]
18. Clement, N.D.; Scott, C.E.; Hamilton, D.F.; MacDonald, D.; Howie, C.R. Meaningful values in the forgotten joint score after total knee arthroplasty: Minimal clinical important difference, minimal important and detectable changes, and patient-acceptable symptom state. *Bone Jt. J.* **2021**, *103*, 846–854. [CrossRef]
19. Murray, D.W.; Fitzpatrick, R.; Rogers, K.; Pandit, H.; Beard, D.J.; Carr, A.J.; Dawson, J. The use of the Oxford hip and knee scores. *J. Bone Jt. Surg. Br.* **2007**, *89*, 1010–1014. [CrossRef]
20. SooHoo, N.F.; Li, Z.; Chenok, K.E.; Bozic, K.J. Responsiveness of patient reported outcome measures in total joint arthroplasty patients. *J Arthroplast.* **2015**, *30*, 176–191. [CrossRef]
21. Cosendey, K.; Eudier, A.; Fleury, N.; Pereira, L.C.; Favre, J.; Jolles, B.M. Ten-year follow-up of a total knee prosthesis combining multi-radius, ultra-congruency, posterior-stabilization and mobile-bearing insert shows long-lasting clinically relevant improvements in pain, stiffness, function and stability. *Knee Surg Sports Traumatol. Arthrosc.* **2023**, *31*, 1043–1052. [CrossRef] [PubMed]
22. Fransen, B.L.; Hoozemans, M.J.M.; Argelo, K.D.S.; Keijser, L.C.M.; Burger, B.J. Fast-track total knee arthroplasty improved clinical and functional outcome in the first 7 days after surgery: A randomized controlled pilot study with 5-year follow-up. *Arch. Orthop. Trauma Surg.* **2018**, *138*, 1305–1316. [CrossRef] [PubMed]
23. Scott, C.E.H.; Bell, K.R.; Ng, R.T.; MacDonald, D.J.; Patton, J.T.; Burnett, R. Excellent 10-year patient-reported outcomes and survival in a single-radius, cruciate-retaining total knee arthroplasty. *Knee Surg Sports Traumatol. Arthrosc.* **2019**, *27*, 1106–1115. [CrossRef]
24. Seetharam, A.; Deckard, E.R.; Ziemba-Davis, M.; Meneghini, R.M. The AAHKS Clinical Research Award: Are Minimum Two-Year Patient-Reported Outcome Measures Necessary for Accurate Assessment of Patient Outcomes after Primary Total Knee Arthroplasty? *J. Arthroplast.* **2022**, *37*, S716–S720. [CrossRef] [PubMed]
25. Berliner, J.L.; Brodke, D.J.; Chan, V.; SooHoo, N.F.; Bozic, K.J. Can Preoperative Patient-reported Outcome Measures Be Used to Predict Meaningful Improvement in Function after TKA? *Clin. Orthop. Relat. Res.* **2017**, *475*, 149–157. [CrossRef] [PubMed]
26. Muertizha, M.; Cai, X.; Ji, B.; Aimaiti, A.; Cao, L. Factors contributing to 1-year dissatisfaction after total knee arthroplasty: A nomogram prediction model. *J. Orthop. Surg. Res.* **2022**, *17*, 367. [CrossRef]
27. Orr, M.N.; Klika, A.K.; Emara, A.K.; Piuzzi, N.S.; Cleveland Clinic Arthroplasty Group. Combinations of Preoperative Patient-Reported Outcome Measure Phenotype (Pain, Function, and Mental Health) Predict Outcome after Total Knee Arthroplasty. *J Arthroplast.* **2022**, *37*, S110–S120.e5. [CrossRef]
28. Elbuluk, A.M.; Jerabek, S.A.; Suhardi, V.J.; Sculco, P.K.; Ast, M.P.; Vigdorchik, J.M. Head-to-Head Comparison of Kinematic Alignment Versus Mechanical Alignment for Total Knee Arthroplasty. *J. Arthroplast.* **2022**, *37*, S849–S851. [CrossRef]
29. MacDessi, S.J.; Oussedik, S.; Abdel, M.P.; Victor, J.; Pagnano, M.W.; Haddad, F.S. The language of knee alignment. *Bone Jt. J.* **2023**, *105*, 102–108. [CrossRef]
30. Vajapey, S.P.; Fitz, W.; Iorio, R. The role of stability and alignment in improving patient outcomes after total knee arthroplasty. *JBJS Rev.* **2022**, *10*, e22. [CrossRef]
31. Dossett, H.G.; Estrada, N.A.; Swartz, G.J.; LeFevre, G.W.; Kwasman, B.G. A randomised controlled trial of kinematically and mechanically aligned total knee replacements: Two-year clinical results. *Bone Jt. J.* **2014**, *96*, 907–913. [CrossRef] [PubMed]
32. Howell, S.M.; Hull, M.L.; Nedopil, A.J.; Riviere, C. Caliper-Verified Kinematically Aligned Total Knee Arthroplasty: Rationale, Targets, Accuracy, Balancing, Implant Survival, and Outcomes. *Instr. Course Lect.* **2023**, *72*, 241–259. [PubMed]
33. Maderbacher, G.; Keshmiri, A.; Krieg, B.; Greimel, F.; Grifka, J.; Baier, C. Kinematic component alignment in total knee arthroplasty leads to better restoration of natural tibiofemoral kinematics compared to mechanic alignment. *Knee Surg Sports Traumatol. Arthrosc.* **2019**, *27*, 1427–1433. [CrossRef] [PubMed]
34. Ettinger, M.; Tsmassiotis, S.; Nedopil, A.J.; Howell, S.M. Calipered technique for kinematic alignment. *Orthopade* **2020**, *49*, 593–596. [CrossRef] [PubMed]
35. Oussedik, S.; Abdel, M.P.; Cross, M.B.; Haddad, F.S. Alignment and fixation in total knee arthroplasty: Changing paradigms. *Bone Jt. J.* **2015**, *97*, 16–19. [CrossRef]
36. Howell, S.M.; Gill, M.; Shelton, T.J.; Nedopil, A.J. Reoperations are few and confined to the most valgus phenotypes 4 years after unrestricted calipered kinematically aligned TKA. *Knee Surg. Sports Traumatol. Arthrosc.* **2021**, *30*, 948–957. [CrossRef]

37. Hollister, A.M.; Jatana, S.; Singh, A.K.; Sullivan, W.W.; Lupichuk, A.G. The axes of rotation of the knee. *Clin. Orthop. Relat. Res.* **1993**, *290*, 259–268. [CrossRef]
38. Clement, N.D.; Bardgett, M.; Weir, D.; Holland, J.; Gerrard, C.; Deehan, D.J. What is the Minimum Clinically Important Difference for the WOMAC Index after TKA? *Clin. Orthop. Relat. Res.* **2018**, *476*, 2005–2014. [CrossRef]
39. Onggo, J.R.; Onggo, J.D.; De Steiger, R.; Hau, R. Robotic-assisted total knee arthroplasty is comparable to conventional total knee arthroplasty: A meta-analysis and systematic review. *Arch. Orthop. Trauma Surg.* **2020**, *140*, 1533–1549. [CrossRef]
40. Zhang, J.; Ndou, W.S.; Ng, N.; Gaston, P.; Simpson, P.M.; Macpherson, G.J.; Patton, J.T.; Clement, N.D. Robotic-arm assisted total knee arthroplasty is associated with improved accuracy and patient reported outcomes: A systematic review and meta-analysis. *Knee Surg. Sports Traumatol. Arthrosc.* **2022**, *30*, 2677–2695. [CrossRef]
41. Huijbregts, H.J.; Khan, R.J.; Sorensen, E.; Fick, D.P.; Haebich, S. Patient-specific instrumentation does not improve radiographic alignment or clinical outcomes after total knee arthroplasty: A meta-analysis. *Acta Orthop.* **2016**, *87*, 386–394. [CrossRef] [PubMed]
42. Ruangsomboon, P.; Ruangsomboon, O.; Pornrattanamaneewong, C.; Narkbunnam, R.; Chareancholvanich, K. Clinical and radiological outcomes of robotic-assisted versus conventional total knee arthroplasty: A systematic review and meta-analysis of randomized controlled trials. *Acta Orthop.* **2023**, *94*, 60–79. [CrossRef] [PubMed]
43. Tandogan, R.N.; Kort, N.P.; Ercin, E.; van Rooij, F.; Nover, L.; Saffarini, M.; Hirschmann, M.T.; Becker, R.; Dejour, D.; European Knee Associates (EKA). Computer-assisted surgery and patient-specific instrumentation improve the accuracy of tibial baseplate rotation in total knee arthroplasty compared to conventional instrumentation: A systematic review and meta-analysis. *Knee Surg. Sports Traumatol. Arthrosc.* **2022**, *30*, 2654–2665. [CrossRef] [PubMed]

**Disclaimer/Publisher's Note:** The statements, opinions and data contained in all publications are solely those of the individual author(s) and contributor(s) and not of MDPI and/or the editor(s). MDPI and/or the editor(s) disclaim responsibility for any injury to people or property resulting from any ideas, methods, instructions or products referred to in the content.

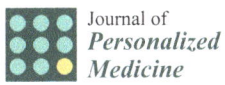

# Journal of Personalized Medicine

*Article*

# Survival of Patient-Specific Unicondylar Knee Replacement

Patrick Weber [1,2,3,*], Melina Beck [1], Michael Klug [4,5], Andreas Klug [4,6], Alexander Klug [4,7], Claudio Glowalla [8] and Hans Gollwitzer [1,2,3,8]

1. ECOM, Arabellastraße 17, 81925 München, Germany
2. ATOS Klinik München, Effnerstraße 38, 81925 München, Germany
3. Dr. Lubos Kliniken München-Bogenhausen, Denninger Straße 44, 81925 München, Germany
4. Knee Centre, Schweinfurter Straße 7, 97080 Würzburg, Germany
5. Praxisklinik Werneck, Balthasar-Neumann-Platz 11-15, 97440 Werneck, Germany
6. König Ludwig Haus, Brettreichstraße 11, 97074 Würzburg, Germany
7. BG Unfallklinik, Friedberger Landstraße 430, 60389 Frankfurt, Germany
8. Klinik und Poliklinik für Orthopädie und Sportorthopädie, Klinikum rechts der Isar, Technische Universität München, Ismaninger Straße 22, 81675 München, Germany
* Correspondence: patrick.weber@atos.de

**Abstract:** Unicompartmental knee arthroplasty (UKA) in isolated medial or lateral osteoarthritis leads to good clinical results. However, revision rates are higher in comparison to total knee arthroplasty (TKA). One reason is suboptimal fitting of conventional off-the-shelf prostheses, and major overhang of the tibial component over the bone has been reported in up to 20% of cases. In this retrospective study, a total of 537 patient-specific UKAs (507 medial prostheses and 30 lateral prostheses) that had been implanted in 3 centers over a period of 10 years were analyzed for survival, with a minimal follow-up of 1 year (range 12 to 129 months). Furthermore, fitting of the UKAs was analyzed on postoperative X-rays, and tibial overhang was quantified. A total of 512 prostheses were available for follow-up (95.3%). Overall survival rate (medial and lateral) of the prostheses after 5 years was 96%. The 30 lateral UKAs showed a survival rate of 100% at 5 years. The tibial overhang of the prosthesis was smaller than 1 mm in 99% of cases. In comparison to the reported results in the literature, our data suggest that the patient-specific implant design used in this study is associated with an excellent midterm survival rate, particularly in the lateral knee compartment, and confirms excellent fitting.

**Keywords:** unicompartmental knee arthroplasty; osteoarthritis; patient-specific implant; partial knee arthroplasty; patient-specific instruments

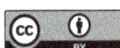

## 1. Introduction

Unicompartmental knee arthroplasty (UKA) in isolated medial or lateral osteoarthritis leads to good clinical results. In comparison to total knee arthroplasty (TKA), surgery can be performed through a shorter approach, leading to quicker rehabilitation, and the kinematics after implantation of UKA are similar to those of the physiological knee [1–4]. Good clinical results were confirmed in two recent randomized controlled trials [5,6]. Registry Data confirmed these results and showed that the Oxford knee score is higher in patients with UKA compared to TKA [7]. On the other hand, the revision rate in UKA is nearly twice as high as for TKA. In the German arthroplasty registry, for example, the revision rate for UKA was 8% after 7 years compared to 4% in TKA [8].

There are many reasons for revision of UKA. The optimal positioning of UKA has been studied extensively [9–11]. In this respect, free-hand implantation of UKA leads to up to 41% of outliers of the optimal range [12]. Other reasons for revision are complications associated with tibial overhang or undersizing. Tibial undersizing may increase the risk of implant migration into the softer cancellous bone with consecutive loosening. On the other hand, a recent analysis showed that a tibial overhang over the bone of more than 3 mm can lead to a revision rate of up to 20% [13]. Medial overhang of the prosthesis is sometimes difficult to avoid. The placement of the medial unicondylar prosthesis is limited in the lateral direction, as harm to the anterior cruciate ligament has to be avoided. Choosing a smaller implant can lead to undercoverage in the antero-posterior direction.

Patient-specific implants (PSI) are produced individually for every patient based on a computed tomography scan of the leg. They have shown a better coverage of the tibia in CAD studies, with 0% overhang in comparison to off-the-shelf implants, which show overhang of up to 70% [14]. Furthermore, it has been shown that the implantation of the PSI in combination with patient-specific instruments leads to reproducible and precise implantation [15]. Thus, PSI should help to avoid suboptimal implantations leading to failures of UKA [12,16].

Lateral UKA can lead to good clinical results in isolated lateral osteoarthritis of the knee [17]. The procedure is performed less frequently and the revision rate is reported to be much higher than in medial UKA, with a revision rate of 12% after 5 years [18]. A reason for this is that lateral UKA is technically more challenging than medial UKA due to the lower number of indications, as well as the different functional anatomy of the lateral compartment. One more reason is the fact that most of the available UKA systems offer no specific lateral implants. Instead, the medial tibial component of one side (left/right) is used as a lateral component on the contralateral side. Knowing that the biomechanics of the lateral component differs to that of the medial, this is probably one reason for the higher revision rate of lateral UKAs [17]. With patient-specific implants a better fitting for lateral prosthesis as well is awaited.

The use of a patient-specific unicompartmental knee prosthesis should result in more precise implantation and better coverage. These advantages should lead to a lower revision rate. However, clinical data showing this are sparse. The aim of this retrospective study was to analyze the survival of more than 500 PSI UKA and to measure the overhang of the tibial component.

## 2. Materials and Methods

A total of 537 consecutive knees in 492 patients that received isolated medial or lateral patient individual UKA (iUni, ConforMIS, Billerica, MA, USA), were included in the study. Surgeries were performed between 09/2010 and 03/2020 in three centers (ECOM Munich, Germany, Knee Centre Würzburg, Germany, and Klinikum rechts der Isar der Technischen Universität München, Germany) by three different surgeons (MK, HG, PW). There were 507 medial prostheses (462 patients) and 30 lateral prostheses (30 patients). Inclusion criteria were patients with anteromedial or lateral osteoarthritis of the knee or avascular osteonecrosis of the medial femoral condyle (AVON, Morbus Ahlbäck) as well as knee pain exclusively localized to the affected compartment.

Exclusion criteria were the following:

- Lateral or medial chondromalacia Grade III or more, or symptomatic retropatellar osteoarthritis
- ROM < Flexion/Extension 100–10–0°
- Varus/Valgus deformity (hip–knee–ankle angle) > 15°
- Patients with valgus knees and medial osteoarthritis or patients with a varus knee in lateral osteoarthritis
- Status after osteotomy
- Ligament insufficiency
- Allergy against metal ions (Ni, Co, Cr)

### 2.1. Prosthesis and Surgical Technique

In all cases, the Conformis iUni knee was implanted. Every patient had a preoperative computed tomography scan of the knee and of the hip and ankle. Planning was performed individually for every patient according to the individual anatomy. The implant was delivered to the surgeon in combination with an iView surgical plan (Figure 1).

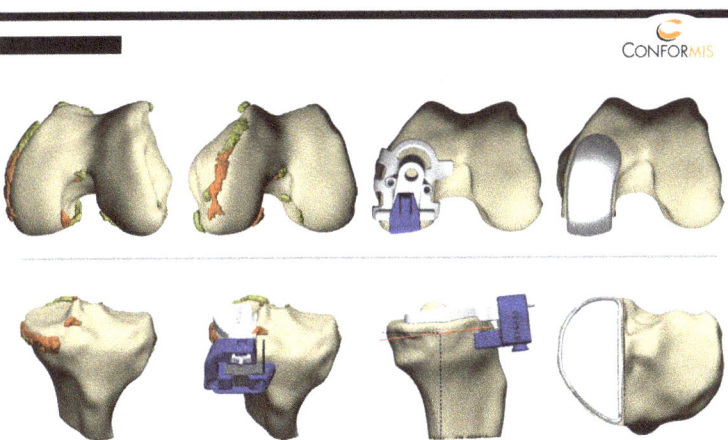

**Figure 1.** Preoperative planning of the prosthesis and surgical guide (Iview) delivered for every patient. It shows the osteophytes that must be removed to position the patient-specific instruments (orange-colored). The position of the patient-specific instruments is also shown. In particular, the position of the femoral jig in accordance with the femoral component is very helpful for the surgeon. Furthermore, it shows the final position of the prosthesis (see further details in the text).

In brief, the prosthesis was implanted for the medial knee through a limited medial parapatellar approach, and for the lateral compartment through a lateral parapatellar arthrotomy. After exposition of the joint and removal of the meniscus, the joint is exposed and isolated medial or lateral osteoarthritis is confirmed. The functional integrity of the anterior cruciate ligament is checked. After this, the rest of the chondral layer on the medial or lateral femoral condyle as well as the osteophytes as indicated on the iView Surgical plan are removed. This step is crucial for correct placement of the individually designed instruments, since the surgical plan is based on the CT scan and therefore on the bony surfaces only. Correct position of the femoral jig (patient-specific instrument) is confirmed by comparison with the surgical plan. The next step consists of removing both the complete remains of the tibial cartilage and the marked osteophytes. Four different heights of balancer chips (1 mm steps) can be inserted into the knee to achieve an appropriate ligament tension. The ligament tension must be appropriate in extension. On the medial side, a laxity of 1–2 mm is aimed on the lateral side of 2–3 mm. After achieving correct ligament tension, the tibial cutting guide is put on the selected balancer chip seating on the tibia. The correct position of the cutting guide is additionally confirmed by an alignment rod attached to the tibia that has to be parallel to the tibial crest. The tibial resection can be performed after fixation of the tibial cutting guide. After removal of the tibial bone, the 8 mm spacer (height of the tibial component and the inlay) is positioned into the knee and the femoral jig is positioned on the femoral bone and in contact with the spacer block. With this technique, the position is achieved in accordance with the bone and the ligament tension. After fixation of the femoral jig, the dorsal femoral resection can be performed. There is no distal femoral resection as the implant is designed to replace only the distal femoral cartilage. Next, the trial is introduced and the joint play is evaluated over the complete range of motion. If satisfactory, the tibial preparation is finished, and the bone is prepared for cementation. Original implants are always cemented with a fixed bearing inlay. If there is excessive joint laxity, a 2-millimeter-higher inlay is available [19].

*2.2. Patient Follow-Up and Data Collection*

All patients are regularly followed-up clinically and radiologically after joint arthroplasty in the three centers (after 6 weeks, 1 year, and then every 2 years). At every control visit, a clinical examination as well as radiography of the knee in two planes are performed.

If patients do not show up to the appointment, they are reminded by phone call. If they cannot come to the appointment, they are asked by phone if the prosthesis is still in situ or if any revision surgery was performed. If patients do not answer, a letter is sent asking them to contact the physicians' office. Revision surgery was defined as exchange arthroplasty of the inlay or the femoral and/or the tibial implant components.

For the study purposes, an evaluation of the patient's charts and already collected data was performed. After all the data were documented for each patient, an irreversible anonymization was undertaken. Ethical approval was obtained prior to the study (Ethikkommission an der Technischen Universität München, Germany, Study 250/21 S-EB). As only a retrospective analysis of already collected data was undertaken with irreversible anonymization, informed consent of the patient was waived by the local ethics committee.

In the study, a minimal follow-up of one year was required. The survival of the prosthesis was assessed, and Kaplan–Meier curves were calculated. A sub-analysis of medial and lateral UKAs was also performed.

Furthermore, antero-posterior respective medial and lateral overhang of the tibial component of the prostheses were measured on the immediate postoperative X-rays.

### 2.3. Statistical Analysis

All statistical analyses were performed using SPSS version 25 (SPSS, Armonk, NY, USA). Descriptive analyses are reported as means, SDs, and ranges for continuous variables, and frequencies and percentages for discrete variables. Overall survivorship was determined using the Kaplan–Meier method.

## 3. Results

### 3.1. Preoperative Data

The preoperative demographic variables of the patients, such as the radiographic state of the osteoarthritis according to the Kellgren and Lawrence classification [20], are shown in Table 1.

**Table 1.** Preoperative characteristics of the patients.

| Variable | Total (n = 537) | Medial UKA (n = 507) | Lateral (n = 30) |
|---|---|---|---|
| Mean age, years (SD) | 66.6 (9.4) | 66.9 (9.9) | 60.9 (9.4) |
| Male sex, n (%) | 313 (58.3) | 299 (59.0) | 16 (53.3) |
| Mean BMI, kg/m² (SD) | 29.2 (4.9) | 29.4 (4.9) [1] | 26.2 (3.6) |
| Preoperative KL [1] grade, n (%) | | | |
| Grade 1 to 2 | 0.2% * | 0.2% | 0 |
| Grade 3 to 4 | 99.8 | 99.8 | 100 |

[1] Kellgren and Lawrence. * Patients with avascular necrosis of the femoral condyle.

### 3.2. Follow-Up

In total, 512 prostheses were available for follow-up (95.3%) at a mean of 4.5 years after surgery (1–10.8 years). Two patients had died (0.2%) and twenty-three (4.5%) were not available for follow-up due to different reasons, such as having disconnected telephone numbers or not answering on multiple attempts. In the patients with medial UKA, the follow-up rate was 95.7% (485/507 patients) at a mean time of 4.6 years (SD 2.4) after surgery. In patients with lateral UKA, the follow-up rate was 90% (27/30 patients) at a mean of 4.2 (SD 2.5) years.

### 3.3. Survival of the Prosthesis

#### 3.3.1. Overall Survival

Survival of the iUni UKA (both lateral and medial) is shown in Figure 2 Overall, survivorship after 4.5 years without revision for any reason was 96.0%.

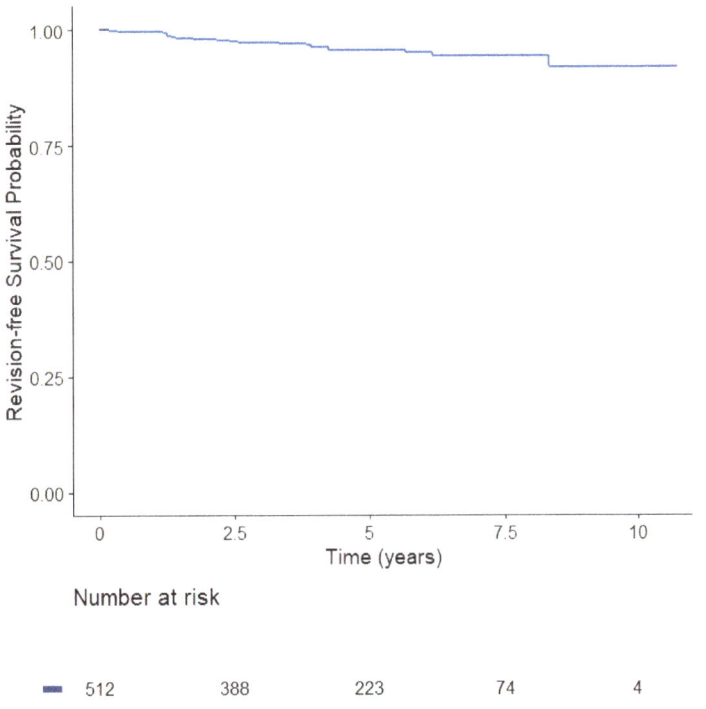

| Time (Years) | Number at Risk | Number of Events | Survival Probability | 95% CI Lower | 95% CI Upper |
|---|---|---|---|---|---|
| All patients, revision for any reason (Figure 2) | | | | | |
| 2 | 417 | 10 | 0.979 | 0.967 | 0.992 |
| 5 | 223 | 8 | 0.955 | 0.935 | 0.976 |
| 10 | 4 | 3 | 0.919 | 0.867 | 0.974 |

**Figure 2.** Kaplan–Meier survival analysis of all patients (512 lateral and medial unicondylar knee prostheses) over time (overall survival with revisions for any reason).

The reasons for revision are given in Table 2.

If only revisions for mechanical failure (aseptic loosening, wear, and periprosthetic fracture) are considered, the survival rate after 4.5 years was 97.5% (Figure 3).

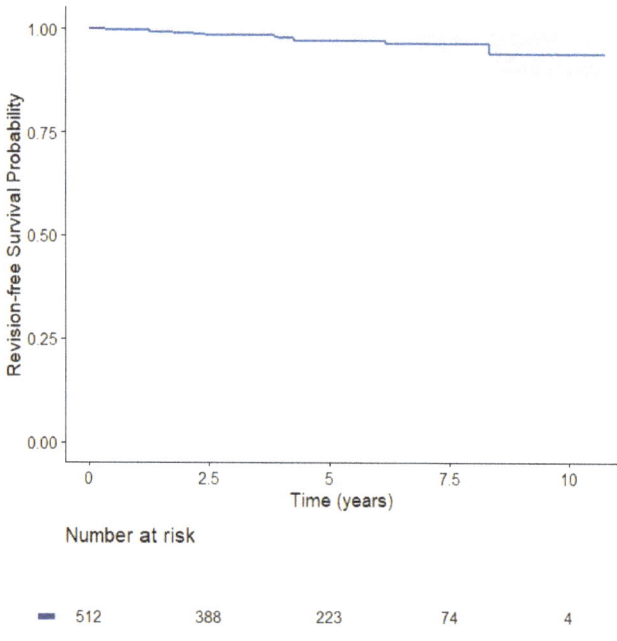

| Time (Years) | Number at Risk | Number of Events | Survival Probability | 95% CI Lower | Upper |
|---|---|---|---|---|---|
| All patients, revision for mechanical reasons (Figure 3) | | | | | |
| 2 | 417 | 5 | 0.989 | 0.980 | 0.999 |
| 5 | 223 | 6 | 0.971 | 0.953 | 0.988 |
| 10 | 4 | 2 | 0.939 | 0.888 | 0.993 |

**Figure 3.** Kaplan–Meier survival analysis of all UKA (512 medial and lateral unicondylar knee prostheses) over time (overall survival with revisions for mechanical reason).

3.3.2. Survival of the Medial UKA

Of the medial UKAs, 20 revisions out of 485 patients were performed after a mean of 4.5 years, corresponding to a survival rate of 95.8% (Figure 4).

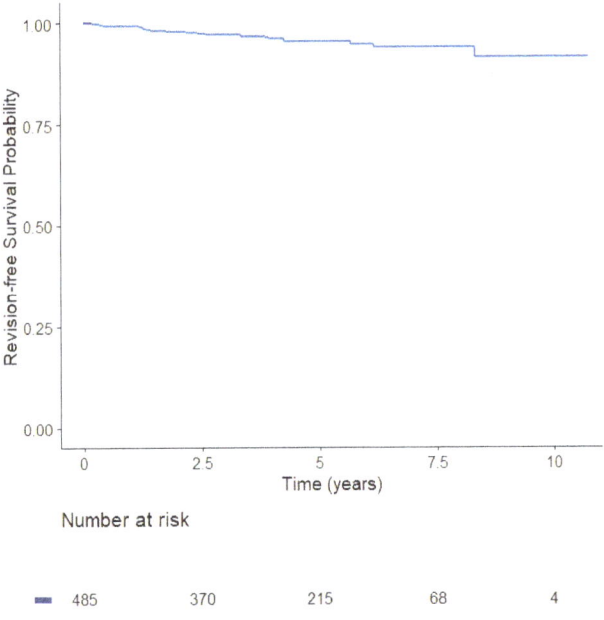

| Time (Years) | Number at Risk | Number of Events | Survival Probability | 95% CI Lower | 95% CI Upper |
|---|---|---|---|---|---|
| Medial only, revision for any reason (Figure 4) | | | | | |
| 2 | 397 | 10 | 0.978 | 0.965 | 0.992 |
| 5 | 215 | 8 | 0.953 | 0.931 | 0.975 |
| 10 | 4 | 3 | 0.915 | 0.860 | 0.973 |

**Figure 4.** Kaplan-Meier survival analysis of the medial UKAs (485 medial unicondylar knee prosthesis) over time (overall survival with revisions for any reason).

### 3.3.3. Survival of the Lateral UKA

The 4.2-year survivorship for the 27 lateral UKAs was 100%. There was no revision of any lateral UKA.

### 3.4. Reasons for Revision

In total, 20 revisions were performed. In nine cases, there was an aseptic loosening leading to revision, and in five cases an infection was the reason for revision. The reasons for revision are displayed in Table 2.

**Table 2.** Reasons for revisions of the iUni arthroplasty (all medial, no revision of lateral knees).

| Reason for Revision | |
|---|---|
| Aseptic loosening (six isolated tibial, three combined femoral + tibial) | 9 (1.73%) |
| Infection | 5 (0.97%) |
| Older periprosthetic fracture | 1 (0.2%) |
| Tibial bone marrow edema | 1 (0.2%) |
| Progressive osteoarthritis in the other compartments | 1 (0.2%) |
| Infrapatellar contracture syndrome (revision at external institution) | 1 (0.2%) |
| Not reported (revision at external institution) | 1 (0.2%) |

*3.5. Radiological Analysis*

Immediate postoperative X-rays were stored in the patient charts and consequently available for work-up in 431 (80.3%) of the 537 initial patients. In four (0.9%) prostheses, there was a medial tibial overhang of up to 3 mm. None had a relevant anteroposterior overhang. Two prostheses (0.5%) had an overhang of 1 mm, one of 2 mm (0.2%), and one of 3 mm (0.2%).

In 404 (79.7%) patients of the medial group, postoperative X-rays were available, with three (0.7%) prostheses showing an overhang of up to 3 mm.

In the lateral group, X-rays were available in all patients. Of these, there was one patient with a lateral overhang of 2 mm (3%).

Figure 5 shows the postoperative X-ray of a lateral UKA:

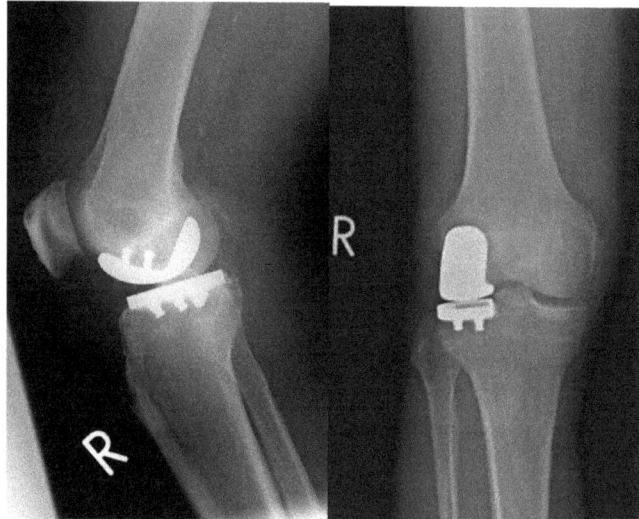

**Figure 5.** Postoperative X-ray of a patient-specific lateral unicondylar knee prosthesis.

## 4. Discussion

The present study evaluated the outcomes of patient-specific UKA for isolated medial or lateral osteoarthritis. Although UKA yields good clinical outcomes, revision rates are relatively high compared to total knee arthroplasty, partly due to poor fitting of conventional off-the-shelf prostheses, resulting in possible overhang of the tibial component over the bone in up to 20% of cases.

This retrospective study analyzed 537 patient-specific UKAs (507 medial and 30 lateral) implanted in three centers over a decade, with a minimal follow-up of 12 months (range: 12–129 months), and is the largest available study on patient-specific UKA. In essence, this study showed a high survival rate in patient-specific unicondylar knee replacement of 96% in 512 knees and of 97% if considering mechanical failure alone at a midterm survival of 4.5 years. Moreover, the theoretical advantage of an excellent fitting of the tibial component of prosthesis to the bone [14] was also shown, with less than 1% of patients showing a tibial overhang of more than 1 mm.

The UKA revision rate is higher compared to TKA. In the most recent report of the German Arthroplasty registry, a revision rate of 7% is reported for UKA after 5 years [8]. In the Australian registry (AAONR), the revision rate at 5 years is comparable with 6.5% and also double the TKA revision rate, which is also the case in the NJR [21,22]. In comparison to these registry data, the present study showed favorable results for an individually designed UKA, with a revision rate of 4% at 5 years. Furthermore, the most impactful data investigating implant survival are currently retrieved from joint replacement registries, since very large numbers can be assessed over time. However, thus far, no registry data have been available for patient-specific UKAs. This emphasizes the importance of performing individual studies with large patient numbers and high follow-up rates. The present study is the largest analysis of the iUni implant, with more than 500 cases involved and a follow-up rate of 95.3%. Thus, the present study is—although limited by its retrospective character—the most robust analysis currently available of implant survival of the patient-specific UKA.

The PSI technique can be compared to modern robotically assisted implantations. A recent study of one center with 1000 knees showed a very high survival rate at 5 years for robotically assisted UKA of 98% excluding inlay exchanges [23]. This survival rate is approximately comparable to the 97% survival rate considering mechanical failure alone observed in this study.

The good survival of the robotically assisted UKA is confirmed in a recent study with data of the Australian registry (AAONR). At 3 years, the robotically assisted UKA had a revision rate of 2.6%, which was half that of the non-robotic UKA (5.0% at 3 years). The best-performing non-robotic UKA reached a revision rate of 3.7% [24]. Again, the PSI of this study showed results comparable to the robotically assisted UKAs and the best non-robotic UKA implant.

There are, to the knowledge of the authors, two studies reporting the results of patient-specific UKA. In the study of Pumilia, 349 knees (same implant as in the present study) were analyzed at a follow-up of 4.8 years with a survival rate of 97.8%, which was slightly better than the results of this study. However, the follow-up rate was less than 70%, which is a potential bias and could have influenced the results [25]. A smaller study also using the iUni by Conformis reported a 100% survival rate of 31 medial UKA after a short-term follow-up of 2.4 years [26].

The present study also included 30 lateral UKAs in 30 patients with a survival rate of 100% at 4.2 years. The lateral compartment of the knee is biomechanically and anatomically different from the medial compartment. Most commercially available unicompartmental implants are not designed specifically for the lateral compartment and therefore the fitting of the prosthesis in the lateral compartment is even more difficult. Furthermore, lateral UKA is performed less frequently, which makes it also more challenging. The literature with follow-up of more than 5 years is sparse, reporting a survival rate of 84–100% for fixed-bearing knees and 79–92% for mobile-bearing knees [27]. The analysis of registry data from the National Joint Registry for England, Wales, Northern Ireland and the Isle of Man revealed 93% survival of 2052 lateral UKAs at 5 years [28]. In contrast, a study by Demange et al., using the same lateral PSI implant also used in the present study, in 33 patients showed a high survival of 97% at 3 years and a better tibial fitting in comparison to a conventional implant. The survival in the conventional group of lateral UKA in the mentioned study was 85% [29]. The present study confirms the favorable results of the PSI, especially in lateral unicompartmental osteoarthritis, in a limited number of patients.

Tibial fitting of the prosthesis is important, as Chau et al. found that an overhang of >3 mm resulted in poorer clinical outcomes on the medial side [30]. In their study, they found an overhang >3 mm in 10% of the patients. Undersizing is also not desirable as the prosthesis will be placed only on weaker cancellous bone, increasing the risk of implant migration and loosening. In a more recent analysis, it was even shown that an overhang of more than 3 mm leads to an increased revision rate of up to 20%, compared to 3% in patients with minor overhang at a follow-up time of five years [13]. The present study showed a very good fitting of patient-specific prostheses, with no overhang of more than 3 mm and only 1% with more than 1 mm. Thus, our study may corroborate the hypothesis that avoidance of tibial overhang is correlated to higher survival rates. The good fitting of the patient-specific tibial component should thus improve survival rate and clinical outcomes.

One possible concern in PSI is the radiation to which patients are exposed through the preoperative computed tomography (CT) scan. Modern CTs have an effective dose between

1 and 7 millisievert (mSv), depending on the organ and the technique. The effective dose for a CT scan of the knee is reported to be 1.3 mSv [31]. In the protocol for PSI, a few slides have to be conducted on the hip joint with a slightly higher dose. The average effective dose through environmental sources is estimated to be 2.4 mSv per year in central Europe, ranging from 1 to 10 mSv depending on activity and the exact living area. Radiation through medical exposures is on average an extra 2 mSv, with variations depending on age and medical condition. The applied radiation of the preoperative CT scan is not negligible. However, it has to be weighed against the potential advantages of PSI. If the implants lead to lower revision rates, there will be reduced radiation for patients that do not need multiple X-rays before and after revision surgery. Furthermore, in conventional knee arthroplasty, preop whole-leg X-ray is mandatory. The radiation of these images is not negligible either. This radiation is not necessary in patients receiving PSI implants, since the leg axis is also determined through CT. Finally, in the opinion of most experts, the risk of developing a disease through CT scanning of the thorax or the abdomen in patients aged over 65 years is negligible [32,33]. Therefore, the much-lower radiation dose of a CT scan of the extremity is probably irrelevant in these patients. Considering the potential advantages of PSI, the necessary radiation for a preoperative CT scan to plan the PSI implants is justifiable in the eyes of the authors.

In spite of the large patient sample, this study has some limitations. First, it was a retrospective analysis with no comparison group. However, it was a consecutive series with a large number of included patients. The follow-up rate of more than 95% is also very high, resulting in a robust data set.

Second, the number of patients receiving a lateral UKA was relatively small. This is due to the significantly rarer indication of lateral UKA. Large case numbers can most likely be obtained with registry analysis, which should also become available for patient-specific implants in the future.

A further limitation of the use of PSI is the costs that are 2–2.5-fold higher than for conventional implants, depending on the country. On the other hand, in PSI there is no need for additional trays, which reduces costs of sterilization and logistics and saves time. If PSI will lead to reduced revisions, as is the case in the present study, there is another potential of saving money by investing more in the implant during primary surgery. In the future, the costs of the implants should also be less by reducing the costs for production through modern 3D printing and an eventually higher use of PSI, which should also reduce costs. Considering all these facts, the costs are probably only slightly higher than in conventional implants, although detailed information of the exact extra costs is missing.

Furthermore, the observed mean follow-up is only 5 years. Nevertheless, it is important to analyze the results at this point also, as eventual advantages or disadvantages of a device and potential risks can already be observed earlier. The present study showed that the survival rate was better in comparison to most of the used UKA at mid-term follow-up, and it is also likely that this difference will be observed in the longer term, justifying continuous use of patient-specific UKA.

Finally, the study does not allow conclusions about the functional results, since no clinical scores were included in the analysis. This has not been the aim of the study, since implant survival should be investigated. There have been many studies showing excellent clinical results in unicompartmental knee replacement [25,26,34], including the implant used in this study. The patients of this study are followed very closely in the centers after UKA, and the low revision rates suggest that the clinical results are also satisfactory. Nevertheless, future studies including clinical results are mandatory.

## 5. Conclusions

The present study is the largest analysis of patient-specific UKA, with more than 500 prostheses analyzed retrospectively. The survival rate of 96% at 4.5 years (97.5% if considering mechanical failure alone) is excellent in comparison to the literature, and comparable to robotic-assisted UKA. Lateral UKA is a more complex procedure with higher risk of revision. The use of a patient-specific implant in this study showed a 100% survival rate at 4.2 years in 30 lateral knees, and these results should be confirmed in the future on a higher number of patients.

**Author Contributions:** conceptualization, P.W., M.B., M.K. and H.G.; methodology, P.W., M.B. and H.G.; investigation P.W., M.B., M.K., A.K. (Andreas Klug), A.K. (Alexander Klug), C.G. and H.G.; writing—original draft preparation, P.W.; writing—review and editing, M.B., M.K., A.K. (Andreas Klug), A.K. (Alexander Klug), C.G. and H.G. All authors have read and agreed to the published version of the manuscript.

**Funding:** This research received no external funding.

**Institutional Review Board Statement:** The study was conducted according to the guidelines of the Declaration of Helsinki, and approved by the Ethics Committee of the Technical University Munich, Germany (250/21 S, 06.07.2021).

**Informed Consent Statement:** Patient consent was waived since no new data were collected, and the analyzed data were irreversibly anonymized. This procedure was chosen after consultation with the local ethics committee.

**Data Availability Statement:** Since this was an observational study, no study registration was undertaken.

**Conflicts of Interest:** The authors declare no conflict of interest.

# References

1. Heyse, T.J.; El-Zayat, B.F.; De Corte, R.; Chevalier, Y.; Scheys, L.; Innocenti, B.; Fuchs-Winkelmann, S.; Labey, L. UKA closely preserves natural knee kinematics in vitro. *Knee Surg. Sport. Traumatol. Arthrosc. Off. J. ESSKA* **2014**, *22*, 1902–1910. [CrossRef] [PubMed]
2. Muller, P.E.; Pellengahr, C.; Witt, M.; Kircher, J.; Refior, H.J.; Jansson, V. Influence of minimally invasive surgery on implant positioning and the functional outcome for medial unicompartmental knee arthroplasty. *J. Arthroplast.* **2004**, *19*, 296–301. [CrossRef] [PubMed]
3. Price, A.J.; Rees, J.L.; Beard, D.J.; Gill, R.H.; Dodd, C.A.; Murray, D.M. Sagittal plane kinematics of a mobile-bearing unicompartmental knee arthroplasty at 10 years: A comparative in vivo fluoroscopic analysis. *J. Arthroplast.* **2004**, *19*, 590–597. [CrossRef] [PubMed]
4. Price, A.J.; Webb, J.; Topf, H.; Dodd, C.A.; Goodfellow, J.W.; Murray, D.W.; Oxford, H.; Knee, G. Rapid recovery after oxford unicompartmental arthroplasty through a short incision. *J. Arthroplast.* **2001**, *16*, 970–976. [CrossRef]
5. Pongcharoen, B.; Liengwattanakol, P.; Boontanapibul, K. Comparison of Functional Recovery Between Unicompartmental and Total Knee Arthroplasty: A Randomized Controlled Trial. *J. Bone Jt. Surg. Am. Vol.* **2023**, *105*, 191–201. [CrossRef]
6. Wu, L.P.; Mayr, H.O.; Zhang, X.; Huang, Y.Q.; Chen, Y.Z.; Li, Y.M. Knee Scores of Patients with Non-Lateral Compartmental Knee Osteoarthritis Undergoing Mobile, Fixed-Bearing Unicompartmental Knee and Total Knee Arthroplasties: A Randomized Controlled Trial. *Orthop. Surg.* **2022**, *14*, 73–87. [CrossRef]
7. Goodfellow, J.W.; O'Connor, J.J.; Murray, D.W. A critique of revision rate as an outcome measure: Re-interpretation of knee joint registry data. *J. Bone Jt. Surg. Br. Vol.* **2010**, *92*, 1628–1631. [CrossRef]
8. EndoprothesenregisterDeutschland. *Jahresbericht 2022*. 2022. Available online: https://www.eprd.de/fileadmin/user_upload/Dateien/Publikationen/Berichte/Jahresbericht2022-Status5_2022-10-25_F.pdf (accessed on 10 January 2023).
9. Weber, P.; Schroder, C.; Schmidutz, F.; Kraxenberger, M.; Utzschneider, S.; Jansson, V.; Muller, P.E. Increase of tibial slope reduces backside wear in medial mobile bearing unicompartmental knee arthroplasty. *Clin. Biomech.* **2013**, *28*, 904–909. [CrossRef]
10. Weber, P.; Schroder, C.; Schwiesau, J.; Utzschneider, S.; Steinbruck, A.; Pietschmann, M.F.; Jansson, V.; Muller, P.E. Increase in the tibial slope reduces wear after medial unicompartmental fixed-bearing arthroplasty of the knee. *Biomed. Res. Int.* **2015**, *2015*, 736826. [CrossRef]
11. Weber, P.; Woiczinski, M.; Steinbruck, A.; Schmidutz, F.; Niethammer, T.; Schroder, C.; Jansson, V.; Muller, P.E. Increase in the Tibial Slope in Unicondylar Knee Replacement: Analysis of the Effect on the Kinematics and Ligaments in a Weight-Bearing Finite Element Model. *Biomed. Res. Int.* **2018**, *2018*, 8743604. [CrossRef]
12. Weber, P.; Crispin, A.; Schmidutz, F.; Utzschneider, S.; Pietschmann, M.F.; Jansson, V.; Muller, P.E. Improved accuracy in computer-assisted unicondylar knee arthroplasty: A meta-analysis. *Knee Surg. Sport. Traumatol. Arthrosc. Off. J. ESSKA* **2013**, *21*, 2453–2461. [CrossRef] [PubMed]
13. Wu, K.; Lv, G.; Yin, P.; Dong, S.; Dai, Z.; Li, L.; Liu, G. Effect of tibial component overhang on survivorship in medial mobile-bearing unicompartmental knee arthroplasty. *Knee* **2022**, *37*, 188–195. [CrossRef] [PubMed]
14. Carpenter, D.P.; Holmberg, R.R.; Quartulli, M.J.; Barnes, C.L. Tibial plateau coverage in UKA: A comparison of patient specific and off-the-shelf implants. *J. Arthroplast.* **2014**, *29*, 1694–1698. [CrossRef] [PubMed]

15. Koeck, F.X.; Beckmann, J.; Luring, C.; Rath, B.; Grifka, J.; Basad, E. Evaluation of implant position and knee alignment after patient-specific unicompartmental knee arthroplasty. *Knee* **2011**, *18*, 294–299. [CrossRef]
16. Hernigou, P.; Deschamps, G. Posterior slope of the tibial implant and the outcome of unicompartmental knee arthroplasty. *J. Bone Jt. Surg. Am.* **2004**, *86*, 506–511. [CrossRef]
17. Ollivier, M.; Abdel, M.P.; Parratte, S.; Argenson, J.N. Lateral unicondylar knee arthroplasty (UKA): Contemporary indications, surgical technique, and results. *Int. Orthop.* **2014**, *38*, 449–455. [CrossRef]
18. Bonanzinga, T.; Tanzi, P.; Altomare, D.; Dorotei, A.; Iacono, F.; Marcacci, M. High survivorship rate and good clinical outcomes at mid-term follow-up for lateral UKA: A systematic literature review. *Knee Surg. Sport. Traumatol. Arthrosc. Off. J. ESSKA* **2021**, *29*, 3262–3271. [CrossRef]
19. Arnholdt, J.; Holzapfel, B.M.; Sefrin, L.; Rudert, M.; Beckmann, J.; Steinert, A.F. Individualized unicondylar knee replacement: Use of patient-specific implants and instruments. *Oper. Orthop. Traumatol.* **2017**, *29*, 31–39. [CrossRef]
20. Kellgren, J.H.; Lawrence, J.S. Radiological assessment of osteo-arthrosis. *Ann. Rheum. Dis.* **1957**, *16*, 494–502. [CrossRef]
21. National_Joint_Registry_for_England_and_Wales. *Report*; 2022; p. 371. Available online: https://reports.njrcentre.org.uk/Portals/0/PDFdownloads/NJR19thAnnualReport2022.pdf (accessed on 10 January 2023).
22. AustralianOrthopaedicAssociationNationalJointReplacementRegistry. *Hip, Knee & Shoulder Arthroplasty 2022 ANNUAL REPORT*; Australian Orthopaedic Association National Joint Replacement Registry: 2022. Available online: https://aoanjrr.sahmri.com/documents/10180/732916/AOA+2022+AR+Digital/f63ed890-36d0-c4b3-2e0b-7b63e2071b16 (accessed on 10 January 2023).
23. Burger, J.A.; Kleeblad, L.J.; Laas, N.; Pearle, A.D. Mid-term survivorship and patient-reported outcomes of robotic-arm assisted partial knee arthroplasty. *Bone Jt. J.* **2020**, *102*, 108–116. [CrossRef]
24. St Mart, J.P.; de Steiger, R.N.; Cuthbert, A.; Donnelly, W. The three-year survivorship of robotically assisted versus non-robotically assisted unicompartmental knee arthroplasty. *Bone Jt. J.* **2020**, *102*, 319–328. [CrossRef] [PubMed]
25. Pumilia, C.A.; Schroeder, L.; Sarpong, N.O.; Martin, G. Patient Satisfaction, Functional Outcomes, and Implant Survivorship in Patients Undergoing Customized Unicompartmental Knee Arthroplasty. *J. Pers. Med.* **2021**, *11*, 753. [CrossRef] [PubMed]
26. Freigang, V.; Rupp, M.; Pfeifer, C.; Worlicek, M.; Radke, S.; Deckelmann, S.; Alt, V.; Baumann, F. Patient-reported outcome after patient-specific unicondylar knee arthroplasty for unicompartmental knee osteoarthritis. *BMC Musculoskelet. Disord.* **2020**, *21*, 773. [CrossRef]
27. Smith, E.; Lee, D.; Masonis, J.; Melvin, J.S. Lateral Unicompartmental Knee Arthroplasty. *JBJS Rev.* **2020**, *8*, e0044. [CrossRef]
28. Baker, P.N.; Jameson, S.S.; Deehan, D.J.; Gregg, P.J.; Porter, M.; Tucker, K. Mid-term equivalent survival of medial and lateral unicondylar knee replacement: An analysis of data from a National Joint Registry. *J. Bone Jt. Surg. Br. Vol.* **2012**, *94*, 1641–1648. [CrossRef] [PubMed]
29. Demange, M.K.; Von Keudell, A.; Probst, C.; Yoshioka, H.; Gomoll, A.H. Patient-specific implants for lateral unicompartmental knee arthroplasty. *Int. Orthop.* **2015**, *39*, 1519–1526. [CrossRef]
30. Chau, R.; Gulati, A.; Pandit, H.; Beard, D.J.; Price, A.J.; Dodd, C.A.; Gill, H.S.; Murray, D.W. Tibial component overhang following unicompartmental knee replacement–does it matter? *Knee* **2009**, *16*, 310–313. [CrossRef]
31. Saltybaeva, N.; Jafari, M.E.; Hupfer, M.; Kalender, W.A. Estimates of effective dose for CT scans of the lower extremities. *Radiology* **2014**, *273*, 153–159. [CrossRef]
32. FDA. What are the Radiation Risks from CT? Available online: https://www.fda.gov/radiation-emitting-products/medical-x-ray-imaging/what-are-radiation-risks-ct (accessed on 19 March 2023).
33. Amis, E.S., Jr.; Butler, P.F.; Applegate, K.E.; Birnbaum, S.B.; Brateman, L.F.; Hevezi, J.M.; Mettler, F.A.; Morin, R.L.; Pentecost, M.J.; Smith, G.G.; et al. American College of Radiology white paper on radiation dose in medicine. *J. Am. Coll. Radiol.* **2007**, *4*, 272–284. [CrossRef]
34. Knifsund, J.; Niinimaki, T.; Nurmi, H.; Toom, A.; Keemu, H.; Laaksonen, I.; Seppanen, M.; Liukas, A.; Pamilo, K.; Vahlberg, T.; et al. Functional results of total-knee arthroplasty versus medial unicompartmental arthroplasty: Two-year results of a randomised, assessor-blinded multicentre trial. *BMJ Open* **2021**, *11*, e046731. [CrossRef]

**Disclaimer/Publisher's Note:** The statements, opinions and data contained in all publications are solely those of the individual author(s) and contributor(s) and not of MDPI and/or the editor(s). MDPI and/or the editor(s) disclaim responsibility for any injury to people or property resulting from any ideas, methods, instructions or products referred to in the content.

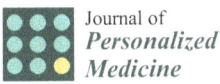

*Review*

# Patient Specific Instruments and Patient Individual Implants—A Narrative Review

Christian Benignus [1], Peter Buschner [2], Malin Kristin Meier [3], Frauke Wilken [2], Johannes Rieger [2] and Johannes Beckmann [2,*]

1. Department of Traumatology and Orthopedic Surgery, Hospital Ludwigsburg, Posilipostr. 4, 71640 Ludwigsburg, Germany
2. Department of Orthopedic Surgery and Traumatology, Hospital Barmherzige Brüder Munich, Romanstr. 93, 80639 Munich, Germany
3. Department of Orthopedic Surgery and Traumatology, Inselspital, University Hospital Bern, University of Bern, Freiburgstr. 4, 3010 Bern, Switzerland
* Correspondence: johannes.beckmann@barmherzige-muenchen.de

**Abstract:** Joint arthroplasties are one of the most frequently performed standard operations worldwide. Patient individual instruments and patient individual implants represent an innovation that must prove its usefulness in further studies. However, promising results are emerging. Those implants seem to be a benefit especially in revision situations. Most experience is available in the field of knee and hip arthroplasty. Patient-specific instruments for the shoulder and upper ankle are much less common. Patient individual implants combine individual cutting blocks and implants, while patient individual instruments solely use individual cutting blocks in combination with off-the-shelf implants. This review summarizes the current data regarding the implantation of individual implants and the use of individual instruments.

**Keywords:** custom-made implants; patient-specific implants; patient-specific instrumentation; Knee arthroplasty; hip arthroplasty; high-tibial osteotomy; kinematic alignment; total ankle arthroplasty; shoulder arthroplasty

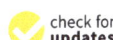

Citation: Benignus, C.; Buschner, P.; Meier, M.K.; Wilken, F.; Rieger, J.; Beckmann, J. Patient Specific Instruments and Patient Individual Implants—A Narrative Review. *J. Pers. Med.* **2023**, *13*, 426. https://doi.org/10.3390/jpm13030426

Academic Editor: Jih-Yang Ko

Received: 13 January 2023
Revised: 20 February 2023
Accepted: 25 February 2023
Published: 27 February 2023

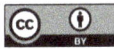

**Copyright:** © 2023 by the authors. Licensee MDPI, Basel, Switzerland. This article is an open access article distributed under the terms and conditions of the Creative Commons Attribution (CC BY) license (https://creativecommons.org/licenses/by/4.0/).

## 1. Introduction

Personalization in medicine is growing enormously and was introduced into orthopaedic surgery several decades ago. Interestingly, one of the first steps was the introduction of robotics in the field of arthroplasty. A large soft-tissue access was required for sufficient exposure. Due to this considerable disadvantage, robotics were banned, but they experienced a renaissance in the last decade [1]. Knee navigation systems were developed in arthroplasty towards the end of the 1990s with the assumption that the accuracy of the prosthesis fit would improve the survival rate of the prosthesis as well as clinical outcomes. The approach via CT-based navigation systems took place for the first time, with imageless systems evolving shortly after. Precision such as leg alignment could significantly be improved by the aid of navigation systems, however, clinical outcome was not. Actual robotic systems are somehow the combination of robots and navigation, again working either CT-based or imageless. Those systems are beyond the topic of this article [2]. In the further course, the broad acquisition of computed tomography (CT) data of bone surfaces was used to produce cutting blocks that would precisely guide the surgeon in the implantation of the prosthesis followed by individual prostheses [3].

These patient-specific implants and instrumentations were launched several years ago to facilitate and improve precise implantation, with the overall aim to improve the outcome of arthroplasty. On the one hand, there is the individual cutting block technology, which is referred to as patient-specific instruments or patient-specific instrumentations. Confusingly, the term patient-specific implants is also used, even though only the cutting blocks are custom-made and standard implants are used for implantation. These are to be distinguished from individual implants, which combine an individual cutting block technology together with individual implants, which can be found in the literature as true patient-specific implants or also as custom-fit or customized implants. Except for total knee arthroplasty, data concerning patient-specific instrumentations are rare, with results often being contradictory but promising. In the last few years, the results, particularly in precision, improved. This might also be attributable to improved scanning and printing technology. These techniques are increasingly used in osteotomies, ankle arthroplasty and shoulder arthroplasty as well as in knee arthroplasty with modern alignment philosophies. Higher costs must be charged up against reduced surgical time, blood loss and fluoroscopic time. Custom-made implants are primarily used, with promising results in hip and knee arthroplasty. Evidence, however, just shows the narrative advantage so far. These primary implants must still prove their effectiveness and superiority in long-term studies before widespread use can be recommended. A growing and clear indication for custom implants, however, is revision situations with bony defects or primary cases with bone deformity.

## 2. Knee Arthroplasty

In contrast to hip arthroplasty, a major problem in knee arthroplasty is the high number of patients who are not satisfied with the results of the operation. Postoperative pain and functional limitations often remain, which in the course of time may lead to prolonged physiotherapeutic measures or even reoperations. This represents a high socio-economic burden. Various factors play a decisive role in patient satisfaction, including the best possible restoration of patient anatomy. The implant design, the surgical technique and also the positioning or the alignment of the prosthesis is crucial in that context [4].

Patient-specific instrumentation (PSI) was introduced into knee arthroplasty roughly two decades ago and comprises the vast majority of the literature. Already, around 2015, there were several systematic reviews that showed no advantage over standard techniques with regard to component alignment as well as clinical outcome [5–8]. However, in the last few years, the results, particularly in precision, improved, which might also be attributable to improved scanning and printing technology. Furthermore, the accuracy of the produced instruments increased by using magnetic resonance imaging (MRI) data rather than CT data. Especially the remaining articular cartilage is hard to be estimated from CT reconstructions. Thus, the cutting blocks may not be able to make sufficient contact with the bony surface. MRI-based cutting blocks offer an easier and more accurate reconstruction in this context. The disadvantage of the MRI technique, however, is the higher susceptibility to motion artefacts. The costs and the extended examination time of the patients must also be considered [9,10]. Thienpont et al. demonstrated in a meta-analysis that the accuracy of femoral component alignment in the coronar plane as well as the global mechanical alignment were significantly improved by PSI. No differences were found with regard to alignment in the axial plane. However, the risk of poorer positioning and malalignment of the tibial component was approximately 30% higher with PSI than for standard instrumentation in both the coronal and sagittal planes [11]. Operative time and blood loss (regardless of calculating as blood volume or hemoglobin count) decreased with the use of the PSI technique compared to standard techniques, but these differences were minimal [11,12]. A more recent study from 2022 showed that tibial rotational positioning can be improved by PSI and that there are fewer outliers compared to conventional techniques [13,14]. Good results with few outliers were also shown for femoral rotational positioning when compared to conventional instrumentation. This is of paramount importance as an incorrect rotation of the femoral component affects the kinematics of the implanted knee prosthesis, possibly resulting in patellar tracking with anterior knee pain, instability and stiffness [15].

Regarding functional outcome, however, still no advantages were found in favor of PSI compared to conventional instrumentation [16,17]. Very interesting is the consideration of costs. A recent retrospective study in the US evaluated total hospital cost and readmission rate at 30, 60, 90, and 365 days in PSI-guided total knee arthroplasty (TKA) patients.

The study matched 3358 TKAs with PSI with TKA-without-PSI patients. Mean total hospital costs were statistically significantly lower for TKA with PSI, at an astonishing USD 14,910 in the US medical system [18]. Another very interesting cost analysis study compared imageless robotics, image-based robotics, navigation and PSI in the medical system of Switzerland. The costs per case were lowest with navigation, comparable between imageless robotics and PSI at roughly USD 1500, and highest with image-based robotics by far.

The most important factors, linked to costs, were technical support and additional disposables. On the contrary, longer surgical times and additional surgical trays only had a minor effect on overall costs [19].

There are conflicting results regarding unicondylar arthroplasty, with each of three papers showing advantages in implantation accuracy [20–22] and no advantages in accuracy nor outcome [23–25], respectively.

With the recent "hot topic debate" of different alignment philosophies, PSI became the further impetus. The PSIs of modern technology could help to implement the plan of kinematic alignment or other novel alignment strategies more precisely. Again, data in the literature are sparse, but they show promising results for PSI with shorter operation times, as well as a lower number of instruments required, and therefore a possible simple and standardized solution for implementing kinematic alignment [26–29].

Individual, custom-made implants (CMI) have been available since 2006, with initially only one company (Conformis, Boston, MA, USA) launching unicondylar implants, which was then chronologically followed by bicompartmental, bicondylar cruciate ligament preserving, and most recently, posterior-stabilized bicondylar implants. A second company manufacturing individual implants has existed for a few years now (Symbios Orthopedie), producing only posterior-stabilized bicondylar implants to date. The main difference between both is the alignment based on the time of the manufacturer's development. While Conformis is aiming for a neutral hip–knee–ankle axis with restoring asymmetry by an oblique joint line (since mechanical alignment was the gold standard in early 2000), Symbios allows a restricted alignment up to 3° in addition to an oblique joint line.

Two recent papers show that CMI have promising results in terms of fit, axis correction, more natural kinematics, patient satisfaction and cost neutrality [30,31]. The Orthopaedic Data Evaluation Panel (ODEP), as an advisory body to the National Health Service (NHS) in the UK, gave Conformis prostheses a 3A rating back in 2017. ODEP draws on data from the National Joint Registry (NJR) for England and Wales as well as expert opinions. Registry data showed a significantly lower early loosening rate for individual implants than for off-the shelf implants. The ODEP believes there is strong evidence of a substantial, patient-relevant improvement in clinical outcomes and a significant reduction in early loosening rates with the individual implant [30]. Meanwhile, the ODEP rating has reached a 7A rating.

On the other hand, neither Moret et al. [31], in a recent literature review, nor Müller et al. [32], in the most recent meta-analysis on total knee arthroplasty (TKA), could find a difference for the clinical outcome between conventional implants and CMI.

In another recent review, the implantation of individualized TKA is not even recommended. It did not demonstrate significant benefits in terms of knee and function scores or range of motion, and had higher early revision rates, although the latter were not statistically significant [33]. Demey et al. also failed to find any advantages in favor of individualized implants in a meta-analysis for partial joint replacement [34]. Higher rates of malpositioning, overcorrection, or loosening were also shown in one study each on TKA, bicompartmental knee arthroplasty (BKA), and unicondylar knee arthroplasty (UKA) [35–37]. However, the promising results of kinematic and biomechanical studies as well as patient-related outcome measurement (PROM) data from various case series suggest decisive improvements in clinical outcomes in favor of CMI [38].

Furthermore, there are three recent comparative studies on the products of both companies, which are mostly not included in meta-analyses. They show clear advantages of CMI compared to off-the shelf implants in terms of pain, mobility, overall outcome, and satisfaction for Conformis (iTotal®) [38–40] as well as Symbios (Origin®), with also very promising clinical and radiological results [41–43]. The latter comparative studies, however, might have conflicting bias as they are at least partly sponsored.

Worldwide, analogously, the number of knee revision surgeries is expected to increase enormously by 601% from 2005 to 2030, solely in the US. Multiple revisions often result in the difficult anchorage of components. Common options for dealing with reduced bone stock after revision surgery, trauma or tumor disease include bulk allografts, impaction grafts, metallic augmentation and porous metal cones/sleeves; however, there are situations where these options reach their limits. Here, CMI (even just the anchoring parts) are increasingly being considered [44]. However, high rates of re-revision occur compared to primary arthroplasty, with complication rates of up to 50% and survival rates of just about 54% after 8 years [45]. These data are based on case reports and small case series due to the inhomogeneity of the patient-specific remaining bone stock.

In summary, PSI shows mixed outcomes for alignment and positioning so far; however, the clear advantages are shorter operation time, reduced blood loss, as well as lower long-term costs. CMI still must prove its value, but the results are very promising.

## 3. Osteotomies

Osteotomies are performed with the aim to correct extra-articular deformities, particularly around the knee, as a pre-arthritic condition in symptomatic patients. The correct analysis of deformities is crucial [46]. Multiplanar deformities exist and are not rare, making either bifocal osteotomies or multiplanar osteotomies necessary, e.g., for the tibia, not just coronal but also sagittal planes (slope) have to be considered.

For this, the angle of correction as well as the sawblade direction are essential.

For preoperative planning, a weight-bearing coronar X-ray of the knee is taken to determine the corrective coronal-plane angle, the size of the osteotomy gap and, if necessary, the screw length [47]. Additionally, a lower-leg X-ray is needed, when multiplanar corrections with additional slope correction have to be addressed.

The standardized positioning of the leg during preoperative and intraoperative X-ray diagnostics is crucial but prone to failure. Measured angles and the range of correction may differ enormously as a result. Likewise, a biplanar correction is difficult to depict with the two-dimensional X-ray procedure and constitutes a further source of error [48]. Here, PSI could clearly assist, being less prone to such failures. However, PSI was introduced to help in several aspects. It can also be used to determine the length and thickness of the plate as well as the length of the necessary screws. This can be prepared preoperatively and thus leads in consequence to a reduction in operation time. The fluoroscopic time can also be reduced compared to conventional osteotomies and the desired correction can be achieved well with the help of PSI [49]. Furthermore, a short learning curve for optimizing an open-wedge high tibial osteotomy using PSI could be demonstrated. The evaluation of the learning curve already showed an advantage in terms of operating time in the first learning phase of the surgeons. In the stable plateau phase of the learning curve, a potential reduction of the operating time to approximately 70% can be assumed compared to the conventional technique [50]. Although good results of the leg axis were shown, there was no significant clinical improvement compared to conventional osteotomies [49–51]. The procedure using PSI also seems to be safe in patients with a pre-operated knee joint. Here, a common previous ACL reconstruction should be mentioned. When planning the osteotomy, the position of the former ACL-drill channels must be taken into account, as well as the hardware inserted. It is essential to avoid the weakening of the inserted ACL reconstruction through the incorrect positioning of the plate or incision [52]. A recent systematic review (of Level-III and -IV studies, however) could confirm a highly accurate coronal plane alignment with a low rate of outliers, significantly shorter operative times and decreased intraoperative fluoroscopy when compared to conventional techniques for both distal femoral as well as proximal tibial osteotomies [53]. Therefore, PSI seems to be a reliable option to facilitate osteotomies and a possible option for pre-operated patients or patients with anatomical norm variants as well. On the other hand, the higher costs of PSI must be weighed up against reduced surgical and fluoroscopic time.

Patient-specific implants obviously have no major role in osteotomies, with well-established plates on the market.

## 4. Shoulder Arthroplasty

In recent years, progress in shoulder arthroplasty has focused in particular on the development of PSI and the further development of inverse shoulder arthroplasty implants and glenoid components, which have gained enormous popularity.

The placement of the glenoid component is often technically challenging and especially difficult in patients who already have significant bone loss at the glenoid due to severe osteoarthritis [54]. Glenoid deformities, as biconcave, retroverted glenoids with humeral subluxation, can often lead to increased complication rates after the implantation of an anatomic prosthesis [55], which is why the implantation of a reverse shoulder prosthesis is often performed in these cases [56]. To better assess the anatomy preoperatively, CT scans are usually performed, from which PSI can also be made. In this way, a target instrument for the glenoid can be manufactured preoperatively, whereby attention must be paid to several parameters such as centering, inclination, anchoring in the bone, and the subluxation of the humeral head [57]. A 2018 meta-analysis of glenoid component implantation in cadavers and humans, comprising 12 studies, showed that deviation from the preoperative planning was significantly lower for the version, inclination and entry point of the pin using PSI compared to standard implants. Furthermore, outliers with a deviation > $10°$ or 4 mm were significantly decreased by PSI (15.3% vs. 68.6%) [58]. However, another meta-analysis from 2019 failed to detect a significant difference between the PSI group and standard implants in terms of version error, inclination error or positional offset. This study described that PSI are expensive to manufacture and take about 6 weeks to be delivered, but they seem to be justified in complicated cases nevertheless [57]. As outsourcing PSI production to external companies is associated with long delivery times and high costs, another study described the use of 3D printers that allow on-site production. The PSI group delivered reliable results; however, only a small case series of cadavers was comprised [59].

Patient-specific implants are not (or not yet?) used in primary arthroplasty but are a good option for patients with complex cases, especially in tumor surgery when large bone resections have to be addressed [60].

However, with the increasing number of primary implantations of artificial shoulder joints, the number of revision operations is also steadily rising. Glenoid loosening and instability of the prosthesis are the most frequent reasons for revision [61]. Due to the pronounced bone loss in the case of replacement operations, the anchoring of the revision prosthesis can be significantly more difficult. Therefore, the need for individual solution strategies in the form of custom-made implants increases. For these cases, some producers offer the production of individual implants from the 3D printer based on 3D-CT or MRI data. Due to the high production costs, however, this is used more individually [57].

In conclusion, the results of the lower deviation in PSI are promising, but the technique is still costly and time-consuming and therefore only considered in individual cases.

## 5. Hip Arthroplasty

PSI in hip surgery will possibly gain influence with osteotomies and have already been introduced into arthroplasty by the guidance of femoral resection as well as cup orientation.

The data concerning custom implants in total hip arthroplasty (THA) are very limited so far and gather around few research centers; however, they have very good results overall. Multicenter, randomized controlled trials and registry data would be desirable to be able to confirm the evidence of the results across the board. Custom implants have been introduced into THA more than two decades ago. Presumably because of the outcome of THA being by far better than in TKA, the manufacturing of customized implants seems to be mainly for special anatomies. It may be especially beneficial for young patients with dysplastic hips. In those patients, standard implants are difficult to implant, but good activity and long survival rates are needed. Only Hitz et al. found a revision rate of 23.1% (six cases) in higher grade dysplasia with, however, good survival rates in terms of the loosening of the stem and cup [62]. Jacquet et al. showed a survival rate of 96.8% after a long-term follow-up of 20 years in a group of patients younger than 50 years and a 96.1% survival rate in those with high-grade developmental dysplasia of the hip, all with good clinical results [63].

The implantation of custom-made cementless stems also seems to be useful after the fusion of the hip joint, with an excellent survival rate and results after 15 years. Flecher et al. examined 23 patients who underwent conversion from a fused hip to THA with a custom femoral implant. Overall, the postoperative complication rate was 26%, which is in line with the literature in this special and rare patient population and included especially heterotopic ossification and aseptic loosening. Conversely, the rate of intra-operative complication was very low, e.g., no intra-operative fracture was observed. It is hypothesized that the use of custom protheses, designed to fit perfectly with the intramedullary anatomy, may explain those differences [64].

In the case of large acetabular bone defects, which are frequently encountered in revision arthroplasty and an enormously growing problem due to increasing numbers of arthroplasties and demographic development itself, standard implants are often inadequate. Bone defects of the acetabulum can be classified according to Paprosky [65] or the American Academy of Orthopedic Surgeons (AAOS), for example [66]. The AAOS classification distinguishes between four different degrees of severity (type I to IV), while Paprosky differentiates six defect types (type I, IIa, IIb, IIc, IIIa, IIIb). If possible, it is better to "down-grade" the defect by means of the biological reconstruction of the acetabular bone. Especially in young, active patients, this can significantly simplify any revision surgery that may occur later. However, the possibility of biological reconstruction is often not sufficient. The overall goal is to restore the center of rotation as well as stability at the acetabular component. At least 50% of the surface of the cementless implant should be covered with autochthonous bone. Types IIIa and IIIb, according to Paprosky, as well as defects according to AAOS types III and IV, are acetabular defects for which different treatment regimens are available with "Jumbo"-cups, pedestal cups or modular options with special augments. Surgical "easiness" as well as defect size caused the desire for a stable monobloc implant that enables defect bridging. This led to the development of individual partial pelvic replacements, especially for the higher-grade defects that are usually associated with instability. The proportion of so-called "mega defects" in acetabular revision cases is given as 1–5% [67]. The available studies in the literature are difficult to compare because the patients' initial situations, prosthesis design and classification of the defects often differ significantly, as does the philosophy of how to reconstruct the defect. Scheele et al. recommend an individual partial pelvic replacement for bone defects that exceed the incisura ischiadica, a non-constructible dorsal rim or pelvic discontinuity [68]. Chiarlone et al. analyzed custom-made implants for large bone defects of the acetabulum in revision total hip arthroplasty in a systematic review and included 634 custom-made acetabular implants (627 patients), with a mean follow-up of $58.6 \pm 29.8$ months from 18 studies. Good clinical and functional results were seen together with a survival rate of $94.0 \pm 5.0$%. Despite this, the re-operation rate was as high as $19.3 \pm 17.3$% and the mean complication rate was $29.0 \pm 16.0$%, with instability being the most common complication [69]. The disadvantage is the high cost of these often-huge custom implants, so they should be used only in special cases, where modular implants cannot be used. The factor time is also important due to the ordering and manufacturing of the implants taking several weeks, during which changes in the patient's bone situation may occur [67]. As has been demonstrated in this paper, custom-made implants show promising clinical results, but considering high costs and long production times, their use has to be judged carefully in every case.

## 6. Total Ankle Arthroplasty (TAA)

The data on PSI TAA are very sparse. There are currently three different types of implants for PSI TAA, two of which are component designs (one talar and one tibial component) and one is a three-component system with a mobile bearing. In a cadaveric study, PSI positioned the implants to less than 2° in all rotational and translational degrees of freedom [70].

Posttraumatic deformities as well as ligament injuries and previous surgeries can make alignment correction more complicated and less predictable. This contrasts with nontraumatic osteoarthritis. Albagli et al. [71] compared the clinical and radiological outcomes of patients with end-stage arthritis—traumatic versus nontraumatic—treated with an implant with CT-guided patient-specific preoperative plans and patient-specific incision patterns. In contrast to previous studies on patients with total ankle arthroplasty in posttraumatic patients, it was shown that there was no difference in patient satisfaction, short-term clinical outcome and radiological outcome when using CT-guided preoperative plans and incision patterns compared to nontraumatic patients. In several studies, the accuracy of implant positioning between the PSI groups and the standard implants was comparable, with no superiority of one group. Patient-specific templates enabled the reproducible positioning of the tibial implant in more than half of the cases, compared to preoperative planning. Discrepancies occurred mainly in severe preoperative varus deformities. In these cases, there are certainly also difficulties in conventional surgery. Postoperative alignment also showed comparable results. The studies were each conducted with experienced surgeons. To what extent an influence exists with inexperienced surgeons could not be shown here [71–75].

The complication and revision rates were comparable after both PSI TAA and the implantation of standard implants [76]. Additionally, the implant size of the tibial component could be estimated quite well using PSI TAA. However, the estimation of the talar component often showed poor results, sometimes less than 50% [76].

After a short follow-up, PSI TAA, using fixed-bearing CT-guided patient-specific implants, showed good results in both traumatic and nontraumatic arthritis compared to standard implants [71]. These results differ from traditional beliefs regarding poorer results with total ankle arthroplasty in posttraumatic patients. Again, surgical time has been shown to be shorter with PSI TAA [74,77], and fluoroscopic time can also be significantly reduced [74]. One study identified a reduction in cost in the PSI group, but this could only be attributed to the reduced surgical time [77]. Further studies with more patients and a longer followup are needed to demonstrate the benefits and theoretical advantages of PSI in TAA.

To date, there have been no studies using patient-specific implants.

## 7. Conclusions

Except for TKA, which is the focus of many studies, data concerning PSI are rare for other indications, with results being contradictory but promising. In the last few years, the results, particularly in precision, have improved, which might also be attributable to improved scanning and printing technology. The usage in osteotomies, ankle arthroplasty and shoulder arthroplasty is growing, which is also true in knee arthroplasty with modern alignment philosophies, which are—talking about kinematic alignment—mostly a compromise of restoring individual anatomy and using symmetric, non-individual implants. Higher costs have to be charged up against reduced surgical time, blood loss and fluoroscopic time. Custom-made implants are primarily used with promising results in hip and knee arthroplasty. The evidence, however, simply shows the narrative advantage so far. These primary implants must still prove their effectiveness and possible superiority in long-term studies before widespread use can be recommended. A growing and clear indication for custom implants, however, is revision situations with bone defects.

**Author Contributions:** Conceptualization, J.B., P.B. and M.K.M.; methodology, C.B., P.B., M.K.M. and J.B.; investigation, C.B., P.B., F.W., J.R. and J.B.; data curation, C.B., F.W. and J.R.; writing—original draft preparation, C.B., P.B., F.W., M.K.M. and J.B.; writing—review and editing, C.B., F.W., J.R. and M.K.M.; visualization, J.R.; supervision, J.B.; project administration, J.B. All authors have read and agreed to the published version of the manuscript.

**Funding:** This research received no external funding.

**Institutional Review Board Statement:** Not applicable.

**Informed Consent Statement:** Not applicable.

**Data Availability Statement:** Not applicable.

**Conflicts of Interest:** The authors declare no conflict of interest.

## References

1. Haaker, R.G.; Tiedjen, K.; Ottersbach, A.; Rubenthaler, F.; Stockheim, M.; Stiehl, J.B. Comparison of conventional versus computer-navigated acetabular component insertion. *J. Arthroplast.* **2007**, *22*, 151–159. [CrossRef]
2. Victor, J.; Van Doninck, D.; Labey, L.; Innocenti, B.; Parizel, P.M.; Bellemans, J. How precise can bony landmarks be determined on a CT scan of the knee? *Knee* **2009**, *16*, 358–365. [CrossRef]
3. Haaker, R. Evolution of total knee arthroplasty. From robotics and navigation to patient-specific instruments. *Orthopade* **2016**, *45*, 280–285. [CrossRef]
4. Ibrahim, M.S.; Khan, M.A.; Nizam, I.; Haddad, F.S. Peri-operative interventions producing better functional outcomes and enhanced recovery following total hip and knee arthroplasty: An evidence-based review. *BMC Med.* **2013**, *11*, 37. [CrossRef]
5. Stronach, B.M.; Pelt, C.E.; Erickson, J.A.; Peters, C.L. Patient-specific instrumentation in total knee arthroplasty provides no improvement in component alignment. *J. Arthroplast.* **2014**, *29*, 1705–1708. [CrossRef]
6. Voleti, P.B.; Hamula, M.J.; Baldwin, K.D.; Lee, G.C. Current data do not support routine use of patient-specific instrumentation in total knee arthroplasty. *J. Arthroplast.* **2014**, *29*, 1709–1712. [CrossRef]
7. Sassoon, A.; Nam, D.; Nunley, R.; Barrack, R. Systematic review of patient-specific instrumentation in total knee arthroplasty: New but not improved. *Clin. Orthop. Relat. Res.* **2015**, *473*, 151–158. [CrossRef]
8. Mannan, A.; Smith, T.O.; Sagar, C.; London, N.J.; Molitor, P.J. No demonstrable benefit for coronal alignment outcomes in PSI knee arthroplasty: A systematic review and meta-analysis. *Orthop. Traumatol. Surg. Res.* **2015**, *101*, 461–468. [CrossRef]
9. Schotanus, M.G.M.; Thijs, E.; Heijmans, M.; Vos, R.; Kort, N.P. Favourable alignment outcomes with MRI-based patient-specific instruments in total knee arthroplasty. *Knee Surg. Sport. Traumatol. Arthrosc. Off. J. ESSKA* **2018**, *26*, 2659–2668. [CrossRef]
10. Wu, X.D.; Xiang, B.Y.; Schotanus, M.G.M.; Liu, Z.H.; Chen, Y.; Huang, W. CT- versus MRI-based patient-specific instrumentation for total knee arthroplasty: A systematic review and meta-analysis. *Surgeon* **2017**, *15*, 336–348. [CrossRef]
11. Thienpont, E.; Schwab, P.E.; Fennema, P. Efficacy of Patient-Specific Instruments in Total Knee Arthroplasty: A Systematic Review and Meta-Analysis. *J. Bone Jt. Surg. Am. Vol.* **2017**, *99*, 521–530. [CrossRef]
12. Lin, Y.; Cai, W.; Xu, B.; Li, J.; Yang, Y.; Pan, X.; Fu, W. Patient-Specific or Conventional Instrumentations: A Meta-analysis of Randomized Controlled Trials. *Biomed. Res. Int.* **2020**, *2020*, 2164371. [CrossRef]
13. Sotozawa, M.; Kumagai, K.; Yamada, S.; Nejima, S.; Inaba, Y. Patient-specific instrumentation for total knee arthroplasty improves reproducibility in the planned rotational positioning of the tibial component. *J. Orthop. Surg. Res.* **2022**, *17*, 403. [CrossRef]
14. Tandogan, R.N.; Kort, N.P.; Ercin, E.; van Rooij, F.; Nover, L.; Saffarini, M.; Hirschmann, M.T.; Becker, R.; Dejour, D. Computer-assisted surgery and patient-specific instrumentation improve the accuracy of tibial baseplate rotation in total knee arthroplasty compared to conventional instrumentation: A systematic review and meta-analysis. *Knee Surg. Sport. Traumatol. Arthrosc. Off. J. ESSKA* **2022**, *30*, 2654–2665. [CrossRef]
15. Mannan, A.; Smith, T.O. Favourable rotational alignment outcomes in PSI knee arthroplasty: A Level 1 systematic review and meta-analysis. *Knee* **2016**, *23*, 186–190. [CrossRef]
16. Rudran, B.; Magill, H.; Ponugoti, N.; Williams, A.; Ball, S. Functional outcomes in patient specific instrumentation vs conventional instrumentation for total knee arthroplasty; a systematic review and meta-analysis of prospective studies. *BMC Musculoskelet. Disord.* **2022**, *23*, 702. [CrossRef]
17. Lei, K.; Liu, L.; Chen, X.; Feng, Q.; Yang, L.; Guo, L. Navigation and robotics improved alignment compared with PSI and conventional instrument, while clinical outcomes were similar in TKA: A network meta-analysis. *Knee Surg. Sport. Traumatol. Arthrosc. Off. J. ESSKA* **2022**, *30*, 721–733. [CrossRef]
18. Thomas, S.; Patel, A.; Patrick, C.; Delhougne, G. Total Hospital Costs and Readmission Rate of Patient-Specific Instrument in Total Knee Arthroplasty Patients. *J. Knee Surg.* **2022**, *35*, 113–121. [CrossRef]
19. Christen, B.; Tanner, L.; Ettinger, M.; Bonnin, M.P.; Koch, P.P.; Calliess, T. Comparative Cost Analysis of Four Different Computer-Assisted Technologies to Implant a Total Knee Arthroplasty over Conventional Instrumentation. *J. Pers. Med.* **2022**, *12*, 184. [CrossRef]

20. Volpi, P.; Prospero, E.; Bait, C.; Cervellin, M.; Quaglia, A.; Redaelli, A.; Denti, M. High accuracy in knee alignment and implant placement in unicompartmental medial knee replacement when using patient-specific instrumentation. *Knee Surg. Sport. Traumatol. Arthrosc. Off. J. ESSKA* **2015**, *23*, 1292–1298. [CrossRef]
21. Kerens, B.; Schotanus, M.G.; Boonen, B.; Kort, N.P. No radiographic difference between patient-specific guiding and conventional Oxford UKA surgery. *Knee Surg. Sport. Traumatol. Arthrosc. Off. J. ESSKA* **2015**, *23*, 1324–1329. [CrossRef]
22. Jones, G.G.; Clarke, S.; Harris, S.; Jaere, M.; Aldalmani, T.; de Klee, P.; Cobb, J.P. A novel patient-specific instrument design can deliver robotic level accuracy in unicompartmental knee arthroplasty. *Knee* **2019**, *26*, 1421–1428. [CrossRef]
23. Ollivier, M.; Parratte, S.; Lunebourg, A.; Viehweger, E.; Argenson, J.N. The John Insall Award: No Functional Benefit After Unicompartmental Knee Arthroplasty Performed with Patient-specific Instrumentation: A Randomized Trial. *Clin. Orthop. Relat. Res.* **2016**, *474*, 60–68. [CrossRef]
24. Li, M.; Zeng, Y.; Wu, Y.; Liu, Y.; Wei, W.; Wu, L.; Peng, B.-q.; Li, J.; Shen, B. Patient-specific instrument for unicompartmental knee arthroplasty does not reduce the outliers in alignment or improve postoperative function: A meta-analysis and systematic review. *Arch. Orthop. Trauma Surg.* **2020**, *140*, 1097–1107. [CrossRef]
25. Leenders, A.M.; Kort, N.P.; Koenraadt, K.L.M.; van Geenen, R.C.I.; Most, J.; Kerens, B.; Boonen, B.; Schotanus, M.G.M. Patient-specific instruments do not show advantage over conventional instruments in unicompartmental knee arthroplasty at 2 year follow-up: A prospective, two-centre, randomised, double-blind, controlled trial. *Knee Surg. Sport. Traumatol. Arthrosc. Off. J. ESSKA* **2022**, *30*, 918–927. [CrossRef]
26. Calliess, T.; Bauer, K.; Stukenborg-Colsman, C.; Windhagen, H.; Budde, S.; Ettinger, M. PSI kinematic versus non-PSI mechanical alignment in total knee arthroplasty: A prospective, randomized study. *Knee Surg. Sport. Traumatol. Arthrosc. Off. J. ESSKA* **2017**, *25*, 1743–1748. [CrossRef]
27. Hommel, H.; Abdel, M.P.; Perka, C. Kinematic femoral alignment with gap balancing and patient-specific instrumentation in total knee arthroplasty: A randomized clinical trial. *Eur. J. Orthop. Surg. Traumatol. Orthop. Traumatol.* **2017**, *27*, 683–688. [CrossRef]
28. Kim, K.K.; Howell, S.M.; Won, Y.Y. Kinematically Aligned Total Knee Arthroplasty with Patient-Specific Instrument. *Yonsei Med. J.* **2020**, *61*, 201–209. [CrossRef]
29. Blakeney, W.G.; Vendittoli, P.-A. Kinematic Alignment Total Knee Replacement with Personalized Instruments. In *Personalized Hip and Knee Joint Replacement*; Rivière, C., Vendittoli, P.-A., Eds.; Springer International Publishing: Cham, Switzerland, 2020; pp. 301–309.
30. Lüring, C.; Beckmann, J. Custom made total knee arthroplasty: Review of current literature. *Orthopade* **2020**, *49*, 382–389. [CrossRef]
31. Moret, C.S.; Schelker, B.L.; Hirschmann, M.T. Clinical and Radiological Outcomes after Knee Arthroplasty with Patient-Specific versus Off-the-Shelf Knee Implants: A Systematic Review. *J. Pers. Med.* **2021**, *11*, 590. [CrossRef]
32. Müller, J.H.; Liebensteiner, M.; Kort, N.; Stirling, P.; Pilot, P.; Demey, G. No significant difference in early clinical outcomes of custom versus off-the-shelf total knee arthroplasty: A systematic review and meta-analysis. *Knee Surg. Sport. Traumatol. Arthrosc. Off. J. ESSKA* **2021**, 1–17. [CrossRef] [PubMed]
33. Beit Ner, E.; Dosani, S.; Biant, L.C.; Tawy, G.F. Custom Implants in TKA Provide No Substantial Benefit in Terms of Outcome Scores, Reoperation Risk, or Mean Alignment: A Systematic Review. *Clin. Orthop. Relat. Res.* **2021**, *479*, 1237–1249. [CrossRef] [PubMed]
34. Demey, G.; Müller, J.H.; Liebensteiner, M.; Pilot, P.; Nover, L.; Kort, N. Insufficient evidence to confirm benefits of custom partial knee arthroplasty: A systematic review. *Knee Surg. Sport. Traumatol. Arthrosc. Off. J. ESSKA* **2022**, *30*, 3968–3982. [CrossRef]
35. Kumar, P.; Elfrink, J.; Daniels, J.P.; Aggarwal, A.; Keeney, J.A. Higher Component Malposition Rates with Patient-Specific Cruciate Retaining TKA than Contemporary Posterior Stabilized TKA. *J. Knee Surg.* **2021**, *34*, 1085–1091. [CrossRef] [PubMed]
36. Talmo, C.T.; Anderson, M.C.; Jia, E.S.; Robbins, C.E.; Rand, J.D.; McKeon, B.P. High Rate of Early Revision After Custom-Made Unicondylar Knee Arthroplasty. *J. Arthroplast.* **2018**, *33*, S100–S104. [CrossRef] [PubMed]
37. Shamdasani, S.; Vogel, N.; Kaelin, R.; Kaim, A.; Arnold, M.P. Relevant changes of leg alignment after customised individually made bicompartmental knee arthroplasty due to overstuffing. *Knee Surg. Sport. Traumatol. Arthrosc. Off. J. ESSKA* **2022**, *30*, 567–573. [CrossRef] [PubMed]
38. Schroeder, L.; Pumilia, C.A.; Sarpong, N.O.; Martin, G. Patient Satisfaction, Functional Outcomes, and Implant Survivorship in Patients Undergoing Customized Cruciate-Retaining TKA. *JBJS Rev.* **2021**, *9*, e20. [CrossRef]
39. Neginhal, V.; Kurtz, W.; Schroeder, L. Patient Satisfaction, Functional Outcomes, and Survivorship in Patients with a Customized Posterior-Stabilized Total Knee Replacement. *JBJS Rev.* **2020**, *8*, e19. [CrossRef]
40. Schroeder, L.; Dunaway, A.; Dunaway, D. A Comparison of Clinical Outcomes and Implant Preference of Patients with Bilateral TKA: One Knee with a Patient-Specific and One Knee with an Off-the-Shelf Implant. *JBJS Rev.* **2022**, *10*, e20. [CrossRef]
41. Bonnin, M.P.; Beckers, L.; Leon, A.; Chauveau, J.; Müller, J.H.; Tibesku, C.O.; Aït-Si-Selmi, T. Custom total knee arthroplasty facilitates restoration of constitutional coronal alignment. *Knee Surg. Sport. Traumatol. Arthrosc. Off. J. ESSKA* **2022**, *30*, 464–475. [CrossRef]
42. Daxhelet, J.; Aït-Si-Selmi, T.; Müller, J.H.; Saffarini, M.; Ratano, S.; Bondoux, L.; Mihov, K.; Bonnin, M.P. Custom TKA enables adequate realignment with minimal ligament release and grants satisfactory outcomes in knees that had prior osteotomies or extra-articular fracture sequelae. *Knee Surg. Sport. Traumatol. Arthrosc. Off. J. ESSKA* **2021**, 1–8. [CrossRef] [PubMed]

43. Ratano, S.; Müller, J.H.; Daxhelet, J.; Beckers, L.; Bondoux, L.; Tibesku, C.O.; Aït-Si-Selmi, T.; Bonnin, M.P. Custom TKA combined with personalised coronal alignment yield improvements that exceed KSS substantial clinical benefits. *Knee Surg. Sport. Traumatol. Arthrosc. Off. J. ESSKA* **2022**, *30*, 2958–2965. [CrossRef] [PubMed]
44. McNamara, C.A.; Gösthe, R.G.; Patel, P.D.; Sanders, K.C.; Huaman, G.; Suarez, J.C. Revision total knee arthroplasty using a custom tantalum implant in a patient following multiple failed revisions. *Arthroplast. Today* **2017**, *3*, 13–17. [CrossRef]
45. Ettinger, M.; Windhagen, H. Individual revision arthroplasty of the knee joint. *Orthopade* **2020**, *49*, 396–402. [CrossRef]
46. Engel, G.M.; Lippert, F.G., 3rd. Valgus tibial osteotomy: Avoiding the pitfalls. *Clin. Orthop. Relat. Res.* **1981**, *160*, 137–143. [CrossRef]
47. Kwun, J.D.; Kim, H.J.; Park, J.; Park, I.H.; Kyung, H.S. Open wedge high tibial osteotomy using three-dimensional printed models: Experimental analysis using porcine bone. *Knee* **2017**, *24*, 16–22. [CrossRef]
48. Kawakami, H.; Sugano, N.; Yonenobu, K.; Yoshikawa, H.; Ochi, T.; Hattori, A.; Suzuki, N. Effects of rotation on measurement of lower limb alignment for knee osteotomy. *J. Orthop. Res.* **2004**, *22*, 1248–1253. [CrossRef]
49. Predescu, V.; Grosu, A.M.; Gherman, I.; Prescura, C.; Hiohi, V.; Deleanu, B. Early experience using patient-specific instrumentation in opening wedge high tibial osteotomy. *Int. Orthop.* **2021**, *45*, 1509–1515. [CrossRef]
50. Jacquet, C.; Sharma, A.; Fabre, M.; Ehlinger, M.; Argenson, J.N.; Parratte, S.; Ollivier, M. Patient-specific high-tibial osteotomy's 'cutting-guides' decrease operating time and the number of fluoroscopic images taken after a Brief Learning Curve. *Knee Surg. Sport. Traumatol. Arthrosc. Off. J. ESSKA* **2020**, *28*, 2854–2862. [CrossRef]
51. Chaouche, S.; Jacquet, C.; Fabre-Aubrespy, M.; Sharma, A.; Argenson, J.N.; Parratte, S.; Ollivier, M. Patient-specific cutting guides for open-wedge high tibial osteotomy: Safety and accuracy analysis of a hundred patients continuous cohort. *Int. Orthop.* **2019**, *43*, 2757–2765. [CrossRef]
52. Jeong, S.H.; Samuel, L.T.; Acuña, A.J.; Kamath, A.F. Patient-specific high tibial osteotomy for varus malalignment: 3D-printed plating technique and review of the literature. *Eur. J. Orthop. Surg. Traumatol. Orthop. Traumatol.* **2022**, *32*, 845–855. [CrossRef] [PubMed]
53. Aman, Z.S.; DePhillipo, N.N.; Peebles, L.A.; Familiari, F.; LaPrade, R.F.; Dekker, T.J. Improved Accuracy of Coronal Alignment Can Be Attained Using 3D-Printed Patient-Specific Instrumentation for Knee Osteotomies: A Systematic Review of Level III and IV Studies. *Arthrosc. J. Arthrosc. Relat. Surg. Off. Publ. Arthrosc. Assoc. N. Am. Int. Arthrosc. Assoc.* **2022**, *38*, 2741–2758. [CrossRef] [PubMed]
54. Dallalana, R.J.; McMahon, R.A.; East, B.; Geraghty, L. Accuracy of patient-specific instrumentation in anatomic and reverse total shoulder arthroplasty. *Int. J. Shoulder Surg.* **2016**, *10*, 59–66. [CrossRef] [PubMed]
55. Denard, P.J.; Walch, G. Current concepts in the surgical management of primary glenohumeral arthritis with a biconcave glenoid. *J. Shoulder Elb. Surg.* **2013**, *22*, 1589–1598. [CrossRef]
56. Mizuno, N.; Denard, P.J.; Raiss, P.; Walch, G. Reverse total shoulder arthroplasty for primary glenohumeral osteoarthritis in patients with a biconcave glenoid. *J. Bone Jt. Surg. Am. Vol.* **2013**, *95*, 1297–1304. [CrossRef] [PubMed]
57. Rolf, O.; Mauch, F. Individualized shoulder arthroplasty: The current state of development. *Orthopade* **2020**, *49*, 424–431. [CrossRef] [PubMed]
58. Villatte, G.; Muller, A.S.; Pereira, B.; Mulliez, A.; Reilly, P.; Emery, R. Use of Patient-Specific Instrumentation (PSI) for glenoid component positioning in shoulder arthroplasty. A systematic review and meta-analysis. *PLoS ONE* **2018**, *13*, e0201759. [CrossRef]
59. Cabarcas, B.C.; Cvetanovich, G.L.; Espinoza-Orias, A.A.; Inoue, N.; Gowd, A.K.; Bernardoni, E.; Verma, N.N. Novel 3-dimensionally printed patient-specific guide improves accuracy compared with standard total shoulder arthroplasty guide: A cadaveric study. *JSES Open Access* **2019**, *3*, 83–92. [CrossRef]
60. Hu, H.; Liu, W.; Zeng, Q.; Wang, S.; Zhang, Z.; Liu, J.; Zhang, Y.; Shao, Z.; Wang, B. The Personalized Shoulder Reconstruction Assisted by 3D Printing Technology After Resection of the Proximal Humerus Tumours. *Cancer Manag. Res.* **2019**, *11*, 10665–10673. [CrossRef]
61. Gauci, M.O.; Cavalier, M.; Gonzalez, J.F.; Holzer, N.; Baring, T.; Walch, G.; Boileau, P. Revision of failed shoulder arthroplasty: Epidemiology, etiology, and surgical options. *J. Shoulder Elb. Surg.* **2020**, *29*, 541–549. [CrossRef]
62. Hitz, O.F.; Flecher, X.; Parratte, S.; Ollivier, M.; Argenson, J.N. Minimum 10-Year Outcome of One-Stage Total Hip Arthroplasty Without Subtrochanteric Osteotomy Using a Cementless Custom Stem for Crowe III and IV Hip Dislocation. *J. Arthroplast.* **2018**, *33*, 2197–2202. [CrossRef] [PubMed]
63. Jacquet, C.; Flecher, X.; Pioger, C.; Fabre-Aubrespy, M.; Ollivier, M.; Argenson, J.N. Long-term results of custom-made femoral stems. *Orthopade* **2020**, *49*, 408–416. [CrossRef]
64. Flecher, X.; Ollivier, M.; Maman, P.; Pesenti, S.; Parratte, S.; Argenson, J.N. Long-term results of custom cementless-stem total hip arthroplasty performed in hip fusion. *Int. Orthop.* **2018**, *42*, 1259–1264. [CrossRef]
65. Paprosky, W.G.; Perona, P.G.; Lawrence, J.M. Acetabular defect classification and surgical reconstruction in revision arthroplasty. A 6-year follow-up evaluation. *J. Arthroplast.* **1994**, *9*, 33–44. [CrossRef]
66. D'Antonio, J.A.; Capello, W.N.; Borden, L.S.; Bargar, W.L.; Bierbaum, B.F.; Boettcher, W.G.; Steinberg, M.E.; Stulberg, S.D.; Wedge, J.H. Classification and management of acetabular abnormalities in total hip arthroplasty. *Clin. Orthop. Relat. Res.* **1989**, *243*, 126–137. [CrossRef]
67. von Lewinski, G. Custom-made acetabular implants in revision total hip arthroplasty. *Orthopade* **2020**, *49*, 417–423. [CrossRef]

68. Scheele, C.; Harrasser, N.; Suren, C.; Pohlig, F.; von Eisenhart-Rothe, R.; Prodinger, P.M. Prospects and challenges of individualized implants in the treatment of large acetabular defects. *OUP* **2018**, *7*, 204–211. [CrossRef]
69. Chiarlone, F.; Zanirato, A.; Cavagnaro, L.; Alessio-Mazzola, M.; Felli, L.; Burastero, G. Acetabular custom-made implants for severe acetabular bone defect in revision total hip arthroplasty: A systematic review of the literature. *Arch. Orthop. Trauma Surg.* **2020**, *140*, 415–424. [CrossRef]
70. Berlet, G.C.; Penner, M.J.; Lancianese, S.; Stemniski, P.M.; Obert, R.M. Total Ankle Arthroplasty Accuracy and Reproducibility Using Preoperative CT Scan-Derived, Patient-Specific Guides. *Foot Ankle Int.* **2014**, *35*, 665–676. [CrossRef]
71. Albagli, A.; Ge, S.M.; Park, P.; Cohen, D.; Epure, L.; Chaytor, R.E.; Volesky, M. Total ankle arthroplasty results using fixed bearing CT-guided patient specific implants in posttraumatic versus nontraumatic arthritis. *Foot Ankle Surg. Off. J. Eur. Soc. Foot Ankle Surg.* **2022**, *28*, 222–228. [CrossRef]
72. Hsu, A.R.; Davis, W.H.; Cohen, B.E.; Jones, C.P.; Ellington, J.K.; Anderson, R.B. Radiographic Outcomes of Preoperative CT Scan-Derived Patient-Specific Total Ankle Arthroplasty. *Foot Ankle Int.* **2015**, *36*, 1163–1169. [CrossRef] [PubMed]
73. Escudero, M.I.; Le, V.; Bemenderfer, T.B.; Barahona, M.; Anderson, R.B.; Davis, H.; Wing, K.J.; Penner, M.J. Total Ankle Arthroplasty Radiographic Alignment Comparison Between Patient-Specific Instrumentation and Standard Instrumentation. *Foot Ankle Int.* **2021**, *42*, 851–858. [CrossRef] [PubMed]
74. Saito, G.H.; Sanders, A.E.; O'Malley, M.J.; Deland, J.T.; Ellis, S.J.; Demetracopoulos, C.A. Accuracy of patient-specific instrumentation in total ankle arthroplasty: A comparative study. *Foot Ankle Surg. Off. J. Eur. Soc. Foot Ankle Surg.* **2019**, *25*, 383–389. [CrossRef]
75. Gagne, O.J.; Veljkovic, A.; Townshend, D.; Younger, A.; Wing, K.J.; Penner, M.J. Intraoperative Assessment of the Axial Rotational Positioning of a Modern Ankle Arthroplasty Tibial Component Using Preoperative Patient-Specific Instrumentation Guidance. *Foot Ankle Int.* **2019**, *40*, 1160–1165. [CrossRef]
76. Wang, Q.; Zhang, N.; Guo, W.; Wang, W.; Zhang, Q. Patient-specific instrumentation (PSI) in total ankle arthroplasty: A systematic review. *Int. Orthop.* **2021**, *45*, 2445–2452. [CrossRef]
77. Hamid, K.S.; Matson, A.P.; Nwachukwu, B.U.; Scott, D.J.; Mather, R.C., 3rd; DeOrio, J.K. Determining the Cost-Savings Threshold and Alignment Accuracy of Patient-Specific Instrumentation in Total Ankle Replacements. *Foot Ankle Int.* **2017**, *38*, 49–57. [CrossRef]

**Disclaimer/Publisher's Note:** The statements, opinions and data contained in all publications are solely those of the individual author(s) and contributor(s) and not of MDPI and/or the editor(s). MDPI and/or the editor(s) disclaim responsibility for any injury to people or property resulting from any ideas, methods, instructions or products referred to in the content.

*Article*

# External Validation of Prediction Models for Surgical Complications in People Considering Total Hip or Knee Arthroplasty Was Successful for Delirium but Not for Surgical Site Infection, Postoperative Bleeding, and Nerve Damage: A Retrospective Cohort Study

Lieke Sweerts [1,2,*], Pepijn W. Dekkers [1], Philip J. van der Wees [2,3], Job L. C. van Susante [4], Lex D. de Jong [4], Thomas J. Hoogeboom [2] and Sebastiaan A. W. van de Groes [1]

1. Department of Orthopaedics, Radboud Institute for Health Sciences, Radboud University Medical Center, 6500 HB Nijmegen, The Netherlands
2. IQ Healthcare, Radboud Institute for Health Sciences, Radboud University Medical Center, 6500 HB Nijmegen, The Netherlands
3. Department of Rehabilitation, Radboud Institute for Health Sciences, Radboud University Medical Center, 6500 HB Nijmegen, The Netherlands
4. Department of Orthopedics, Rijnstate Hospital, 6800 TA Arnhem, The Netherlands
* Correspondence: lieke.sweerts@radboudumc.nl

**Abstract:** Although several models for the prediction of surgical complications after primary total hip or total knee replacement (THA and TKA, respectively) are available, only a few models have been externally validated. The aim of this study was to externally validate four previously developed models for the prediction of surgical complications in people considering primary THA or TKA. We included 2614 patients who underwent primary THA or TKA in secondary care between 2017 and 2020. Individual predicted probabilities of the risk for surgical complication per outcome (i.e., surgical site infection, postoperative bleeding, delirium, and nerve damage) were calculated for each model. The discriminative performance of patients with and without the outcome was assessed with the area under the receiver operating characteristic curve (AUC), and predictive performance was assessed with calibration plots. The predicted risk for all models varied between <0.01 and 33.5%. Good discriminative performance was found for the model for delirium with an AUC of 84% (95% CI of 0.82–0.87). For all other outcomes, poor discriminative performance was found; 55% (95% CI of 0.52–0.58) for the model for surgical site infection, 61% (95% CI of 0.59–0.64) for the model for postoperative bleeding, and 57% (95% CI of 0.53–0.61) for the model for nerve damage. Calibration of the model for delirium was moderate, resulting in an underestimation of the actual probability between 2 and 6%, and exceeding 8%. Calibration of all other models was poor. Our external validation of four internally validated prediction models for surgical complications after THA and TKA demonstrated a lack of predictive accuracy when applied in another Dutch hospital population, with the exception of the model for delirium. This model included age, the presence of a heart disease, and the presence of a disease of the central nervous system as predictor variables. We recommend that clinicians use this simple and straightforward delirium model during preoperative counselling, shared decision-making, and early delirium precautionary interventions.

**Keywords:** decision support techniques; external validation; prediction; surgical complications; total hip arthroplasty; total knee arthroplasty

## 1. Introduction

Discussing the risk of surgical complications with patients is an important part of shared decision-making in patients with end-stage hip or knee osteoarthritis considering total hip or knee arthroplasty (THA or TKA). Previous research demonstrates that surgical complications are associated with factors relating to demography, comorbidities, and medication use [1], and that these factors combined might predict the risk of surgical complications [2–5]. Prediction models provide an estimate of a patient's preoperative risk by calculating individual predicted probabilities for surgical complications, and can thereby be used to facilitate preoperative personalized counselling and shared decision-making.

Although several prediction models for preoperative counselling regarding the risk of surgical complications are available [2,4–15], only two studies validated these models externally for patients considering primary THA and TKA [3,16]. External validation is important because differences in, for example, population characteristics and setting may affect the applicability of the prediction models in another hospital population [17]. The available studies that did evaluate the external validation of preoperative prediction models regarding the risk of surgical complications after THA and TKA found moderate-to-poor predictive performance in a new context and patient population, rendering these models unfit for application in clinical practice [3,16]. These results emphasize the need for further research in the development of accurate risk stratification tools specified for people opting for THA or TKA.

Only three studies with three procedure-specific prediction models to predict the risk on a surgical site infection after primary THA or TKA have been published [2,14,15], and to our knowledge, none of these models have been externally validated [18]. Focusing upon one of these studies, our own research group recently published a set of easy to use and potentially valid prediction models [2]. These prediction models have been developed specifically for the preoperative counselling of four surgical complications: surgical site infection, postoperative bleeding, delirium, and nerve damage after primary THA and TKA. These four models are considered to have good applicability since the models comprised less than eight predictor variables, which is considered easy to use in clinical practice [19]. Furthermore, the models in this study showed moderate-to-good discriminative capacity, and are considered to be valuable in predicting these surgical complaints since current counselling is based on population-based risks [19]. However, these models were only validated internally on the basis of data from a single academic hospital setting in the Netherlands [2], which generally is a setting which includes a more complex patient population. Furthermore, the applicability of the models has not yet been confirmed using data of patients from another setting, and the models' predictive performance using a non-academic hospital population has not been tested. In other words, the performance of these prediction models in an external population is unknown; this is important to determine whether the models are transferrable to a broader context. The aim of this study was to determine the external validity of four previously developed models for surgical complications in people considering primary THA or TKA surgery by determining the predictive performance in this new context.

## 2. Materials and Methods

### 2.1. Study Design, Setting, and Population

In this retrospective cohort study, four prediction models developed previously by Sweerts et al. were externally validated using data from a cohort of patients from Rijnstate Hospital in Arnhem, the Netherlands [2]. We considered this cohort as being representative of a non-academic hospital population in the Netherlands. The prediction models were originally developed for patients considering primary THA or TKA. As such, patients for our current study were eligible for inclusion if they had had a THA or TKA for the first time. Patients who had revision arthroplasty of one or several components of the joint prosthesis were excluded because research has shown that revision surgery increases the risk for surgical complications [2,20,21].

All patients that underwent primary THA or TKA between 2017 and 2020 and met the inclusion criteria were contacted to ask for their consent to use their pseudonymized patient data.

Approval for this study was granted by the Institutional Research Board of Rijnstate Hospital (2020-1584). The study was performed and reported in line with transparent reporting of a multivariable prediction model for individual prognosis or diagnosis (TRIPOD-) guidelines [22].

*2.2. Data Extraction and Handling*

Data of variables used in the prediction models were extracted from the patients' electronic health records using CTcue, a self-service data mining tool with text-mining features (CTcue, v4.4.1; Amsterdam, The Netherlands, www.ctcue.com, accessed on 12 July 2022). This clinical data collection tool is powered by artificial intelligence and machine learning to parse, structure, and interpret data. The tool adheres to the General Data Protection Regulation and the program uses pseudo-identification to ensure patient privacy [23]. Identifiers that could be linked to individual patients (e.g., names, addresses, phone numbers) were pseudonymized. The tool was used to extract both structured (e.g., age, measurement values, standardized diagnostic codes, test results) and unstructured (free texts such as the physician's medical notes and evaluations) patient data from electronic health record systems by use of a query. The query used in this study was based on specification of the category to extract data from the electronic health record, and was further specified by filtering on specific report type, period, specialism, date, etc. A variety of categories of the electronic health record system can be searched as reports, medication administrations, appointments, care activities, surgeries, vital signs, etc. [23]. The program collates these data in an analyzable dataset [23]. Data were extracted by combining keywords with commonly known synonyms, variants, abbreviations, and frequent typographical errors as suggested by the application programming interface. One researcher (LS) created the query and checked all the extracted data using the validation tool of the clinical data collection tool. The query for this study was initially performed with high sensitivity. The query was later narrowed while checking whether this would not lead to any data loss. The query was fine-tuned to the point where no new information was found. The query used can be found in Supplementary Materials Table S1. Structured data were considered missing if the outcome variable was not available from the patients' electronic health record. These missing data were first checked for patterns of randomness, and subsequently imputed by multiple imputation, using predictive mean matching. The number of imputations was set to ten. The imputation was checked for accuracy by visual inspection and frequencies. Specific outcome variables not reported in the unstructured data (e.g., no comments about infections or comorbid conditions in the free text fields) were considered as a sign that these were also not present in that particular patient. After the search using CTcue, another researcher (PD) extracted all relevant data from the electronic health records manually. Both researchers subsequently randomly checked the accuracy of 100 patient records by comparing the clinical data collection tool and manual data extraction. The agreement between the automated and manual search was measured by Cohen's κ coefficient, with κ = 0.41–0.60 indicating moderate agreement, κ = 0.61–0.80 representing good agreement, and κ ≥ 0.81 representing very good agreement [24].

*2.3. Predictor Variables*

In line with the previously developed models, we extracted the following variables: age, gender, BMI, smoking status (yes/no), the presence of predefined comorbidities (yes/no), and predefined medication use (yes/no) [2]. Comorbidities included the presence of an immunological disorder, rheumatoid arthritis, diabetes mellitus, liver disease, heart disease, disease of the central nervous system, and/or hip dysplasia. Information collected regarding medication use included the of use of vitamin K antagonists, and/or non-steroid anti-inflammatory drugs (NSAID) [2].

## 2.4. Predictor Variables

The outcome variables used for the external validation of the prediction models included the presence (yes/no) of surgical site infection within 90 days after surgery, postoperative bleeding, delirium and nerve damage [2]. Only models with a mean AUC >0.7 in the developmental phase were considered appropriate for external validation. Therefore, the models for venous thromboembolism and luxation were not included in this study.

## 2.5. Sample Size

The sample size was based on the rule of thumb that at least five events per variable are required for each predictor in the models [25]. An event was defined as the postoperative occurrence of one of the predefined surgical complications. In the Netherlands, the risk of a surgical complication such as surgical site infection is 3% [26]. As the prediction model for surgical site infection consists of six variables, a sample size of at least 1000 patients was required ($6 \times 5/0.03 = 1000$).

## 2.6. Data Analysis
### 2.6.1. Predicted Probabilities

To validate the prediction models, for each patient an individual predicted probability was calculated by integrating the following linear part prediction formulas developed by Sweerts et al., in $1/(1 + \exp^{-\text{linear part}}) \times 100\%$ [2]:

1. Surgical site infection: $-7.272 + (0.031 \times \text{age} - 0.002 \times \text{BMI} + 0.757 \times \text{smoking status} + 0.891 \times \text{immunological disorder} + 0.904 \times \text{diabetes mellitus} + 2.345 \times \text{liver disease} + 0.619 \times \text{NSAID's})$;
2. Postoperative bleeding: $-7.172 + (0.033 \times \text{age} + 0.012 \times \text{BMI} - 0.023 \times \text{smoking status} + 0.729 \times \text{heart disease} + 0.787 \times \text{vitamin K antagonist use})$;
3. Delirium: $-14.307 + (0.127 \times \text{age} + 0.348 \times \text{heart disease} + 0.898 \times \text{disease of central nervous system})$;
4. Nerve damage: $-2.250 + (-0.051 \times \text{age} - 0.254 \times \text{gender} + 0.572 \times \text{smoking status} - 0.009 \times \text{dysplasia})$.

### 2.6.2. Predicted Probabilities

The overall model performance was expressed by the distance between the predicted and actual outcome [27]. To quantify model performance, the Brier statistic was determined. For the Brier statistic, squared differences between the actual outcome and predictions were calculated. The Brier statistic can range from 0 for a perfect model to 0.25 for a non-informative model with 50% incidence of the outcome [28]. The ability of the model to discriminate between patients with and without the outcome was assessed using the area under the curve (AUC). The AUC can range from 50% (no discriminative capacity) to 100% (perfect discriminative capacity). The discriminative capacity was considered moderate when AUC was > 0.70 and good when AUC was > 0.80 [29]. Calibration of the model is the agreement between predicted probabilities (probability of an event calculated with the model) and observed frequencies of outcome (accuracy) and was assessed by visually inspecting the calibration plot [27]. Furthermore, we computed Hosmer and Lemeshow (H-L) goodness-of-fit as a quantitative measure of calibration. A high H-L statistic is related to a low $p$-value, and indicates a poor fit [30]. All statistical analyses were performed using R 3.5.3 and its extension packages vim, mice, rms, pROC, and generalhoslem [31].

## 3. Results

A total of 2641 medical records of patients who received THA or TKA were included. Of these, 1407 patients received a primary THA and 1207 patients received a primary TKA.

Patient characteristics of the study cohort are shown in Table 1. The mean age was 68 years and 62% of the patients were female.

Table 1. Patient characteristics of study cohort.

| Patient Characteristics | Missing Values | Total Cohort (n = 2614) | Patients after THA (n = 1407) | Patients after TKA (n = 1207) |
|---|---|---|---|---|
| Age (years, mean ± SD) | 0% | 68.1 ± 10 | 68.8 ± 10.5 | 67.4 ± 9.4 |
| Gender: female (n, %) | 0% | 1628 (62.3) | 892 (63.4) | 736 (61) |
| BMI (mean ± SD) | 1.20% | 28.8 ± 5 | 27.7 ± 4.8 | 30.1 ± 5.1 |
| Smoking: yes (n, %) | 1.30% | 522 (20) | 304 (21.9) | 218 (18.2) |
| Surgical complications (n, %) | | | | |
| -surgical site infection | 0% | 38 (1.5) | 23 (1.6) | 15 (1.2) |
| -postoperative bleeding | 0% | 74 (2.8) | 40 (2.8) | 34 (2.8) |
| -delirium | 0% | 21 (0.8) | 8 (0.6) | 13 (1.1) |
| -nerve damage | 0% | - | 2 (0.1) | - |
| Comorbidities (n, %) | | | | |
| -immunological disorder | 0% | 316 (12.1) | 152 (10.8) | 164 (13.6) |
| -rheumatoid arthritis | 0% | 205 (7.8) | 101 (7.2) | 104 (8.6) |
| -diabetes mellitus | 0% | 348 (13.3) | 159 (11.3) | 189 (15.7) |
| -liver disease | 0% | 41 (1.6) | 24 (1.7) | 17 (1.4) |
| -heart disease | 0% | 622 (23.8) | 342 (24.3) | 280 (23.2) |
| -disease of central nervous system | 0% | 145 (5.5) | 76 (5.4) | 69 (5.7) |
| -hip dysplasia | 0% | 39 (1.5) | 36 (2.6) | 3 (0.2) |
| Medication use | | | | |
| -vitamin K antagonist | 0% | 151 (5.8) | 87 (6.2) | 64 (5.3) |
| -NSAID | 0% | 296 (11.3) | 189 (13.4) | 107 (8.9) |

Abbreviations: BMI, body mass index; NSAID, non-steroid anti-inflammatory drugs.

The automated versus manual search resulted in an agreement of κ = 0.94 for the extraction of the structured data. A κ = 0.55 was found for the extraction of the unstructured data.

### 3.1. Model Development

The number of missing values per predictor variable is shown in Table 1. For the majority of the predictors, there were no missing data. Missing data were found for BMI (1.2%) and smoking status (1.3%). Analysis showed that the data were missing at random. After multiple imputation, all data of all patients were available for analysis.

### 3.2. Model Performance

The ROC curves representing the discriminative performance of the prediction models are shown in Figure 1. The corresponding AUCs are reported in Table 2.

Table 2. Discriminative (AUC) and predictive (H-L) performance per model.

| Discriminative and Predictive Performance | Area under the Curve (AUC) (95%CI) | H-L Statistic (p-Value) |
|---|---|---|
| Surgical site infection | 0.55 (0.52–0.58) | <0.001 |
| Postoperative bleeding | 0.61 (0.59–0.64) | <0.001 |
| Delirium | 0.84 (0.82–0.87) | <0.001 |
| Nerve damage | 0.57 (0.53–0.61) | <0.001 |

Abbreviations: AUC, area under the curve: the ability to discriminate between those with and without the outcome. The AUC can range from 0.50 (no discriminative capacity) to 1.00 (perfect discriminative capacity). H-L statistic, Hosmer and Lemeshow: quantitative measure of calibration. High H-L statistic is related to a low p-Value and indicates a poor fit.

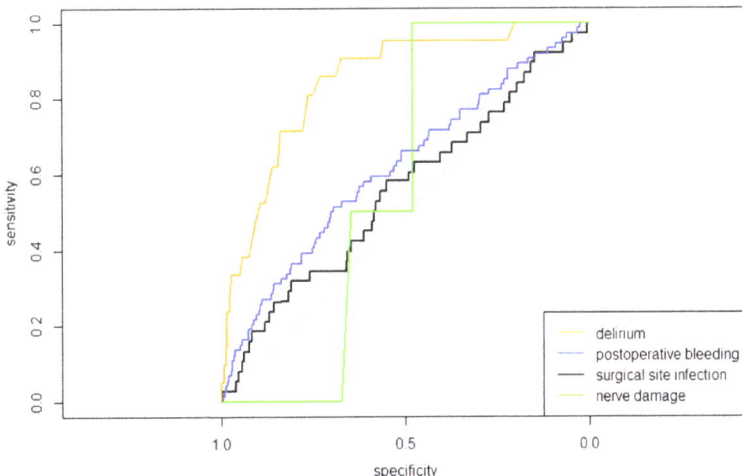

**Figure 1.** ROC curves of all four models predicting surgical complications, indicating the discriminative performance of all models concerning the probability of a surgical complication.

The mean predicted probability for surgical site infection was 1.3% (range 0.2–33.5%). For postoperative bleeding, delirium, and nerve damage, the mean predicted probabilities of, respectively, 1.5% (range 0.2–8.6%), 0.8% (range 0.01–11.8%), and 0.3% (range 0.05–4.1%) were found, see also Table 3. The predictive performances of the models are shown in the calibration plots in Supplementary Materials Figure S1. The model for surgical site infection showed an overestimation exceeding 2% risk for surgical site infection. The model for postoperative bleeding showed an underestimation of the actual risk, and the model for nerve damage showed poor calibration overall. For delirium, moderate calibration was found, resulting in an underestimation of the actual probability between 2 and 6% and exceeding 8%. The H-L statistic showed $p$-Values < 0.001 for all models, which indicates a poor fit.

**Table 3.** Mean predicted risk, and Brier statistic per model.

| Overall Performance | Mean Predicted Risk % (SD) | Brier Statistic |
| --- | --- | --- |
| Surgical site infection | 0.013 (0.022) Range 0.002–0.335 | 0.015 |
| Postoperative bleeding | 0.015 (0.012) Range 0.002–0.086 | 0.028 |
| Delirium | 0.008 (0.011) Range <0.001–0.118 | 0.008 |
| Nerve damage | 0.003 (0.003) Range 0.001–0.041 | 0.001 |

Brier statistic: to quantify model performance. Squared differences between actual outcome and predictions are calculated. The score can range from 0 for a perfect model to 0.25 for a non-informative model with 50% incidence of the outcome [27].

## 4. Discussion

The aim of this study was to externally validate four previously developed models for preoperative counselling by predicting the risk for surgical site infection, postoperative bleeding, delirium, and nerve damage in patients after THA and TKA. External validation showed only good performance for delirium. Calibration of the model for delirium was acceptable, and the discriminative capacity was good with an AUC 95%-lower limit confidence interval of 0.82. For all other models, calibration was poor, resulting in under- or overestimation, and discriminative capacity was poor to moderate. The results for the models for surgical site infection, postoperative bleeding, and nerve damage showed diminished accuracy when used on another population than originally developed for, and do not provide reliable estimations of the predicted probabilities to be used in preoperative counselling and shared decision-making. Overall, external validation showed a loss of discriminative performance; the original AUC for the model for surgical site infection was 72% instead of 55% for the model in external validation. The same corresponds for postoperative bleeding; 73% vs. 61%, delirium; 86% vs. 84%, and nerve damage; 77% vs. 57% [2].

Only three studies with three procedure-specific prediction models (including the models which we externally validated in this study) to predict surgical site infection are available in the literature for comparison with our results [2,14,15]. To our knowledge, these procedure-specific models have not been externally validated previously [18]. For a prediction of postoperative bleeding, delirium, and nerve damage, no other procedure-specific models for preoperative counselling in THA or TKA have been found.

Previous research has shown that the external validation of prediction models often results in poorer performance [32], and that external validation using different populations is negatively influenced by differences in centers (geographical validation) [33]. The same may have been true for this external validation. The differences in patients between the cohorts of the academic and non-academic hospitals may have led to the poor results for the prediction of surgical site infection, postoperative bleeding, and nerve damage.

The model of delirium showed moderate discriminative capacity with three included predictors. Only this model was found to be appropriate for clinical use and we consider this result important for preoperative counselling and shared decision-making. The model consists of three predictor variables only (age, heart disease, and disease of central nervous system), and as such, may be easy to use since the predictors are considered to be known in usual preoperative care. Being able to predict postoperative delirium based on three predictor variables is arguably useful in clinical practice to take early precautions to prevent or treat delirium.

All in all, a plethora of prediction models for the prediction of surgical complications are available—universal models, procedure-specific models, models with many variables, and models with a smaller amount of variables—but a common problem is that numerous models after external validation seem to have difficulties regarding discrimination and calibration and thereby clinical applicability to (another) specific population [34]. In this case, it can be recommended to adjust or recalibrate a model for local circumstances by the use of information of the primary model with information of the validation study [34,35].

*Strengths and Limitations*

We used a reproducible, automated method to extract the data from the electronic health records, and we cross-checked the automated search with a manual search. The cross-check revealed very good agreement between the automated and manual extraction of the structured data ($\kappa = 0.94$). A moderate agreement ($\kappa = 0.55$) was found for the data extraction of the unstructured data. Checking the results showed that the automated search with the clinical data collection tool extracted the unstructured data more accurately than the researcher because the former was searching in more sources (e.g., medical notes and evaluations reported by all medical specialists within a predefined timeframe) while the manual extraction was limited to orthopedic and preoperative anesthesia data. Additionally, we selected a representative cohort of patients, as shown by the comparable frequencies of postoperative complications within our (academic hospital) reference cohort and the current (non-academic hospital) cohort.

This study has a number of limitations. We collected retrospective data using a clinical data collection tool. This tool is considered a promising tool for retrieving real-world data from electronic health records because relevant outcome data can be identified [36]. However, data extracted from this system only represent (real-world) data that are entered in the electronic patient records. If these latter data are incomplete, erroneous, or missing, they will also (negatively) influence the retrieved data. For example, we found several typographical errors in the physicians' notes and different physicians used different terminology for the same diseases; this will arguably have negatively influenced the data extractions. On the other hand, the clinical data collection tool assisted in mitigating these issues by proposing a combination of keywords, commonly known synonyms, word variations, abbreviations, common typographical errors, and by checking data for accuracy using a built-in validation tool. Furthermore, we tried to prevent discrepancies and errors by employing a sensitive search first and specifying the query by adding information while continuously confirming that no data loss took place. Although we tried to prevent errors with multiple activities, we cannot rule out having missed registered comorbidities in text fields, which may have resulted in an underestimation of the frequencies of comorbidities. Another limitation is our low number of events regarding the surgical outcomes, particularly for nerve damage. We cannot ensure this to be of influence on the results of this external validation, especially regarding model calibration. Different to other studies, the model for delirium did not include smoking status and gender as predictor candidates for the prediction of delirium; this is in contrast with other studies [37,38]. In the developmental study, predictor candidates were selected based on evidence from the literature, clinical reasoning, and eyeballing potential higher frequencies in the data [2]. The chosen method of inclusion has not led to the inclusion of these potential predictors based on the developmental cohort.

## 5. Conclusions

This study externally validated four prediction models that are aimed to improve preoperative counselling and shared decision-making at the orthopedics department. Only the model for delirium showed good discriminative capacity and calibration to be appropriate for clinical use. The results for the models for surgical site infection, postoperative bleeding, and nerve damage suggest that these models do not provide sufficient predictive accuracy to be applied in clinical settings. Taking the effective ways to prevent and/or threaten delirium into account, we expect the model for the prediction of delirium to be valuable for preoperative counselling, shared decision-making, and early delirium precautionary interventions. This expectation is strengthened by the fact that this model included only age, the preoperative presence of a heart disease, and the presence of a disease of the central nervous system as predictor variables, thus encompassing the proven important ease of use by keeping the data entry to a minimum [19]. Studies assessing the utility of these models are needed to explore if these prediction models can improve counselling efforts and have practical benefits.

**Supplementary Materials:** The following supporting information can be downloaded at: https://www.mdpi.com/article/10.3390/jpm13020277/s1, Supplementary Materials Table S1: Query CTcue; Supplementary Materials Figure S1: Calibration plot per surgical complication indicating the calibration of the models.

**Author Contributions:** Conceptualization, L.S., P.J.v.d.W., T.J.H. and S.A.W.v.d.G.; methodology, L.S., P.J.v.d.W., J.L.C.v.S., L.D.d.J., T.J.H. and S.A.W.v.d.G.; software, not applicable; validation, L.S. and P.W.D.; formal analysis, L.S. and P.W.D.; investigation, L.S.; resources, P.J.v.d.W., J.L.C.v.S., L.D.d.J., T.J.H. and S.A.W.v.d.G.; data curation, L.S. and P.W.D.; writing—original draft preparation, L.S.; writing—review and editing, P.W.D., P.J.v.d.W., J.L.C.v.S., L.D.d.J., T.J.H. and S.A.W.v.d.G.; visualization, L.S.; supervision, P.J.v.d.W., J.L.C.v.S., L.D.d.J., T.J.H. and S.A.W.v.d.G.; project administration, L.S.; funding acquisition, not applicable. All authors have read and agreed to the published version of the manuscript.

**Funding:** This research received no external funding.

**Institutional Review Board Statement:** The study was conducted in accordance with the Declaration of Helsinki, and approved by the Institutional Review Board (or Ethics Committee) of Rijnstate Hospital (2020-1584; 1 July 2020).

**Informed Consent Statement:** Informed consent was obtained from all subjects involved in the study.

**Data Availability Statement:** Data are available upon reasonable request.

**Conflicts of Interest:** Philip van der Wees participates in the Scientific Advisory Panel of the American Physical Therapy Association (APTA). All other authors declare no conflicts of interest.

## References

1. Podmore, B.; Hutchings, A.; van der Meulen, J.; Aggarwal, A.; Konan, S. Impact of comorbid conditions on outcomes of hip and knee replacement surgery: A systematic review and meta-analysis. *BMJ Open* **2018**, *8*, e021784. [CrossRef] [PubMed]
2. Sweerts, L.; Hoogeboom, T.J.; van Wessel, T.; van der Wees, P.J.; van de Groes, S.A.W. Development of prediction models for complications after primary total hip and knee arthroplasty: A single-centre retrospective cohort study in the Netherlands. *BMJ Open* **2022**, *12*, e062345. [CrossRef]
3. Trickey, A.W.; Ding, Q.; Harris, A.H.S. How Accurate Are the Surgical Risk Preoperative Assessment System (SURPAS) Universal Calculators in Total Joint Arthroplasty? *Clin. Orthop. Relat. Res.* **2020**, *478*, 241–251. [CrossRef] [PubMed]
4. Harris, A.H.S.; Kuo, A.C.; Weng, Y.; Trickey, A.W.; Bowe, T.; Giori, N.J. Can Machine Learning Methods Produce Accurate and Easy-to-use Prediction Models of 30-day Complications and Mortality After Knee or Hip Arthroplasty? *Clin. Orthop. Relat. Res.* **2019**, *477*, 452–460. [CrossRef] [PubMed]
5. Harris, A.H.; Kuo, A.C.; Bowe, T.; Gupta, S.; Nordin, D.; Giori, N.J. Prediction Models for 30-Day Mortality and Complications After Total Knee and Hip Arthroplasties for Veteran Health Administration Patients with Osteoarthritis. *J. Arthroplast.* **2018**, *33*, 1539–1545. [CrossRef]
6. Bilimoria, K.Y.; Liu, Y.; Paruch, J.L.; Zhou, L.; Kmiecik, T.E.; Ko, C.Y.; Cohen, M.E. Development and evaluation of the universal ACS NSQIP surgical risk calculator: A decision aid and informed consent tool for patients and surgeons. *J. Am. Coll. Surg.* **2013**, *217*, 833–842.e831–833. [CrossRef]
7. Protopapa, K.L.; Simpson, J.C.; Smith, N.C.; Moonesinghe, S.R. Development and validation of the Surgical Outcome Risk Tool (SORT). *Br. J. Surg.* **2014**, *101*, 1774–1783. [CrossRef] [PubMed]
8. Meguid, R.A.; Bronsert, M.R.; Juarez-Colunga, E.; Hammermeister, K.E.; Henderson, W.G. Surgical Risk Preoperative Assessment System (SURPAS): III. Accurate Preoperative Prediction of 8 Adverse Outcomes Using 8 Predictor Variables. *Ann. Surg.* **2016**, *264*, 23–31. [CrossRef] [PubMed]
9. Bozic, K.J.; Ong, K.; Lau, E.; Berry, D.J.; Vail, T.P.; Kurtz, S.M.; Rubash, H.E. Estimating risk in Medicare patients with THA: An electronic risk calculator for periprosthetic joint infection and mortality. *Clin. Orthop. Relat. Res.* **2013**, *471*, 574–583. [CrossRef]
10. Tan, T.L.; Maltenfort, M.G.; Chen, A.F.; Shahi, A.; Higuera, C.A.; Siqueira, M.; Parvizi, J. Development and Evaluation of a Preoperative Risk Calculator for Periprosthetic Joint Infection Following Total Joint Arthroplasty. *JBJS* **2018**, *100*, 777–785. [CrossRef] [PubMed]
11. Zotov, E.; Hills, A.F.; de Mello, F.L.; Aram, P.; Sayers, A.; Blom, A.W.; McCloskey, E.V.; Wilkinson, J.M.; Kadirkamanathan, V. JointCalc: A web-based personalised patient decision support tool for joint replacement. *Int. J. Med. Inform.* **2020**, *142*, 104217. [CrossRef] [PubMed]
12. Paxton, E.W.; Inacio, M.C.S.; Khatod, M.; Yue, E.; Funahashi, T.; Barber, T. Risk Calculators Predict Failures of Knee and Hip Arthroplasties: Findings from a Large Health Maintenance Organization. *Clin. Orthop. Relat. Res.* **2015**, *473*, 3965–3973. [CrossRef] [PubMed]
13. Klemt, C.; Tirumala, V.; Smith, E.J.; Padmanabha, A.; Kwon, Y.-M. Development of a Preoperative Risk Calculator for Reinfection Following Revision Surgery for Periprosthetic Joint Infection. *J. Arthroplast.* **2021**, *36*, 693–699. [CrossRef] [PubMed]
14. Everhart, J.S.; Andridge, R.R.; Scharschmidt, T.J.; Mayerson, J.L.; Glassman, A.H.; Lemeshow, S. Development and Validation of a Preoperative Surgical Site Infection Risk Score for Primary or Revision Knee and Hip Arthroplasty. *JBJS* **2016**, *98*, 1522–1532. [CrossRef] [PubMed]
15. Inacio, M.C.S.; Pratt, N.L.; Roughead, E.E.; Graves, S.E. Predicting Infections After Total Joint Arthroplasty Using a Prescription Based Comorbidity Measure. *J. Arthroplast.* **2015**, *30*, 1692–1698. [CrossRef]
16. Edelstein, A.I.; Kwasny, M.J.; Suleiman, L.I.; Khakhkhar, R.H.; Moore, M.A.; Beal, M.D.; Manning, D.W. Can the American College of Surgeons Risk Calculator Predict 30-Day Complications After Knee and Hip Arthroplasty? *J. Arthroplast.* **2015**, *30*, 5–10. [CrossRef]
17. Steyerberg, E.W.; Moons, K.G.; van der Windt, D.A.; Hayden, J.A.; Perel, P.; Schroter, S.; Riley, R.D.; Hemingway, H.; Altman, D.G. Prognosis Research Strategy (PROGRESS) 3: Prognostic model research. *PLoS Med.* **2013**, *10*, e1001381. [CrossRef]
18. Kunutsor, S.K.; Whitehouse, M.R.; Blom, A.W.; Beswick, A.D. Systematic review of risk prediction scores for surgical site infection or periprosthetic joint infection following joint arthroplasty. *Epidemiol. Infect.* **2017**, *145*, 1738–1749. [CrossRef]
19. Kilsdonk, E.; Peute, L.W.; Jaspers, M.W.M. Factors influencing implementation success of guideline-based clinical decision support systems: A systematic review and gaps analysis. *Int. J. Med. Inform.* **2017**, *98*, 56–64. [CrossRef]
20. Ong, K.L.; Lau, E.; Suggs, J.; Kurtz, S.M.; Manley, M.T. Risk of Subsequent Revision after Primary and Revision Total Joint Arthroplasty. *Clin. Orthop. Relat. Res.* **2010**, *468*, 3070–3076. [CrossRef]
21. Van Steenbergen, L.N.; Denissen, G.A.W.; Spooren, A.; van Rooden, S.M.; van Oosterhout, F.J.; Morrenhof, J.W.; Nelissen, R.G.H.H. More than 95% completeness of reported procedures in the population-based Dutch Arthroplasty Register. *Acta Orthop.* **2015**, *86*, 498–505. [CrossRef] [PubMed]

22. Moons, K.G.; Altman, D.G.; Reitsma, J.B.; Ioannidis, J.P.; Macaskill, P.; Steyerberg, E.W.; Vickers, A.J.; Ransohoff, D.F.; Collins, G.S. Transparent Reporting of a multivariable prediction model for Individual Prognosis or Diagnosis (TRIPOD): Explanation and elaboration. *Ann. Intern. Med.* **2015**, *162*, W1–W73. [CrossRef] [PubMed]
23. CTcue. Empowering Healthcare with Real-World Evidence. Available online: https://ctcue.com/ (accessed on 12 July 2022).
24. Landis, J.R.; Koch, G.G. The measurement of observer agreement for categorical data. *Biometrics* **1977**, *33*, 159–174. [CrossRef] [PubMed]
25. Vittinghoff, E.; McCulloch, C.E. Relaxing the rule of ten events per variable in logistic and Cox regression. *Am. J. Epidemiol.* **2007**, *165*, 710–718. [CrossRef] [PubMed]
26. Van Arkel, E.; van der Kraan, J.; Hageman, M.; Venhorst, K. Consultkaart Artrose in de heup. 2016. Available online: https://cdn.nimbu.io/s/yba55wt/assets/20161219_CK_Artrose-in-de-heup.pdf (accessed on 12 July 2022).
27. Steyerberg, E.W. *Clinical Prediction Models*; Springer: New York, NY, USA, 2009.
28. Steyerberg, E.W.; Vickers, A.J.; Cook, N.R.; Gerds, T.; Gonen, M.; Obuchowski, N.; Pencina, M.J.; Kattan, M.W. Assessing the performance of prediction models: A framework for traditional and novel measures. *Epidemiology* **2010**, *21*, 128–138. [CrossRef] [PubMed]
29. Hosmer, D.W.; Lemeshow, S.; Sturdivant, R. *Applied Logistic Regression*, 3rd ed.; Wiley: New York, NY, USA, 2013.
30. Peduzzi, P.; Concato, J.; Kemper, E.; Holford, T.R.; Feinstein, A.R. A simulation study of the number of events per variable in logistic regression analysis. *J. Clin. Epidemiol.* **1996**, *49*, 1373–1379. [CrossRef] [PubMed]
31. R Development Core Team. R: A language and environment for statistical computing, R Foundation for Statistical Computing. 2010. Available online: http://www.R-project.org (accessed on 27 July 2022).
32. Siontis, G.C.; Tzoulaki, I.; Castaldi, P.J.; Ioannidis, J.P. External validation of new risk prediction models is infrequent and reveals worse prognostic discrimination. *J. Clin. Epidemiol.* **2015**, *68*, 25–34. [CrossRef]
33. Wynants, L.; Collins, G.S.; Van Calster, B. Key steps and common pitfalls in developing and validating risk models. *BJOG* **2017**, *124*, 423–432. [CrossRef]
34. Shipe, M.E.; Deppen, S.A.; Farjah, F.; Grogan, E.L. Developing prediction models for clinical use using logistic regression: An overview. *J. Thorac. Dis.* **2019**, *11*, S574–S584. [CrossRef]
35. Moons, K.G.; Kengne, A.P.; Grobbee, D.E.; Royston, P.; Vergouwe, Y.; Altman, D.G.; Woodward, M. Risk prediction models: II. External validation, model updating, and impact assessment. *Heart* **2012**, *98*, 691–698. [CrossRef]
36. Van Laar, S.A.; Gombert-Handoko, K.B.; Guchelaar, H.-J.; Zwaveling, J. An Electronic Health Record Text Mining Tool to Collect Real-World Drug Treatment Outcomes: A Validation Study in Patients with Metastatic Renal Cell Carcinoma. *Clin. Pharmacol. Ther.* **2020**, *108*, 644–652. [CrossRef] [PubMed]
37. Nandi, S.; Harvey, W.F.; Saillant, J.; Kazakin, A.; Talmo, C.; Bono, J. Pharmacologic Risk Factors for Post-Operative Delirium in Total Joint Arthroplasty Patients: A Case–Control Study. *J. Arthroplast.* **2014**, *29*, 268–271. [CrossRef] [PubMed]
38. Kitsis, P.; Zisimou, T.; Gkiatas, I.; Kostas-Agnantis, I.; Gelalis, I.; Korompilias, A.; Pakos, E. Postoperative Delirium and Postoperative Cognitive Dysfunction in Patients with Elective Hip or Knee Arthroplasty: A Narrative Review of the Literature. *Life* **2022**, *12*, 314. [CrossRef] [PubMed]

**Disclaimer/Publisher's Note:** The statements, opinions and data contained in all publications are solely those of the individual author(s) and contributor(s) and not of MDPI and/or the editor(s). MDPI and/or the editor(s) disclaim responsibility for any injury to people or property resulting from any ideas, methods, instructions or products referred to in the content.

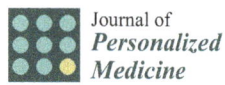 

Article

# A Deep Learning Method for Quantification of Femoral Head Necrosis Based on Routine Hip MRI for Improved Surgical Decision Making

Adrian C. Ruckli [1,†], Andreas K. Nanavati [2,*,†], Malin K. Meier [2], Till D. Lerch [3], Simon D. Steppacher [2], Sébastian Vuilleumier [2], Adam Boschung [4], Nicolas Vuillemin [2], Moritz Tannast [4], Klaus A. Siebenrock [2], Nicolas Gerber [1] and Florian Schmaranzer [3]

1. Personalised Medicine Research, School of Biomedical and Precision Engineering, University of Bern, 3008 Bern, Switzerland
2. Department of Orthopaedic Surgery and Traumatology, Inselspital, University Hospital of Bern, 3010 Bern, Switzerland
3. Department of Diagnostic-, Interventional- and Pediatric Radiology, Inselspital, University Hospital of Bern, 3010 Bern, Switzerland
4. Department of Orthopaedic Surgery and Traumatology, Fribourg Cantonal Hospital, University of Fribourg, 1752 Fribourg, Switzerland
* Correspondence: akn40@case.edu; Tel.: +41-79-560-28-19, Postal Code: 07043
† These authors contributed equally to this work.

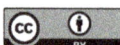

**Abstract:** (1) *Background*: To evaluate the performance of a deep learning model to automatically segment femoral head necrosis (FHN) based on a standard 2D MRI sequence compared to manual segmentations for 3D quantification of FHN. (2) *Methods*: Twenty-six patients (thirty hips) with avascular necrosis underwent preoperative MR arthrography including a coronal 2D PD-w sequence and a 3D T1 VIBE sequence. Manual ground truth segmentations of the necrotic and unaffected bone were then performed by an expert reader to train a self-configuring nnU-Net model. Testing of the network performance was performed using a 5-fold cross-validation and Dice coefficients were calculated. In addition, performance across the three segmentations were compared using six parameters: volume of necrosis, volume of unaffected bone, percent of necrotic bone volume, surface of necrotic bone, unaffected femoral head surface, and percent of necrotic femoral head surface area. (3) *Results*: Comparison between the manual 3D and manual 2D segmentations as well as 2D with the automatic model yielded significant, strong correlations ($R_p > 0.9$) across all six parameters of necrosis. Dice coefficients between manual- and automated 2D segmentations of necrotic- and unaffected bone were 75 ± 15% and 91 ± 5%, respectively. None of the six parameters of FHN differed between the manual and automated 2D segmentations and showed strong correlations ($R_p > 0.9$). Necrotic volume and surface area showed significant differences (all $p < 0.05$) between early and advanced ARCO grading as opposed to the modified Kerboul angle, which was comparable between both groups ($p > 0.05$). (4) *Conclusions*: Our deep learning model to automatically segment femoral necrosis based on a routine hip MRI was highly accurate. Coupled with improved quantification for volume and surface area, as opposed to 2D angles, staging and course of treatment can become better tailored to patients with varying degrees of AVN.

**Keywords:** hip; femoral head necrosis; Kerboul angle; MRI; segmentation; deep learning

## 1. Introduction

Femoral head necrosis (FHN) is a significant cause of hip osteoarthritis and a disabling disease of the hip, particularly in young adults [1]. Once osteonecrosis is apparent through radiographic or clinical evidence, arthritis and collapse of the femoral head will likely occur without any subsequent intervention [2]. In fact, FHN has been shown to account for roughly 10% of all total hip arthroplasties along with 10,000 to 20,000 new cases annually in the United States alone [3]. In Asia and sub-Saharan Africa, the burden is even worse, with over 50% of total hip replacements performed being attributed to FHN [4].

Prognosis for FHN depends on the presence of a subchondral fracture of the bone, coupled with the location, size of the necrotic lesions, and stage of the disease [5]. In most cases, patients display large, necrotic lesions accompanied by femoral head fragmentation, with progression to end-stage osteoarthritis in 2–3 years. However, even smaller lesions with an intact femoral head can progress to subcortical fractures and femoral collapse, taking place in up to 50% of cases [6]. Especially problematic is the early introduction of hip prostheses in younger patients, where their higher activity levels limit the prosthetic's durability, requiring multiple implant changes later on [7]. Alternative procedures to joint replacement for FHN include core decompression and vascularized bone grafting, which look to restore the blood supply to the femoral head [8,9]. Others include femoral osteotomies, which aim to reposition necrotic bone away from the weightbearing portion of the joint [10], and surgical hip dislocations, which provide access to the entire joint and have shown promising results for the treatment of more advanced FHN [5,11].

Despite these options, there is no consensus for the optimal course of action for FHN, nor in which patients with FHN will rapidly progress and whom will need surgical treatment to obviate this [6]. Currently, the revised ARCO classification, along with the Kerboul angle (used to estimate the extent of necrosis), can help prognosticate FHN [12], but these are limited to radiographs and 2D MR images. With the Kerboul angle in particular, the assessment of the size and location crucial for the grading is only semiquantitative, relying on indirect assessment and eyeballing. To date, there remains no tried and tested method to directly quantify the volume of necrosis relative to healthy bone, nor to measure the necrotic surface area in the weight bearing zone of the femoral head to incorporate into the staging [13]. This makes it very difficult to standardize surgical decision making for FHN due to the lack of rigorous evaluation and high observer-dependence [13,14].

Although staging for FHN is based on 2D imaging techniques, high-resolution 3D MRI sequences, along with the necessary graphic processing units and development of novel machine-learning based applications, should enable reconstruction of 3D MRI-based models for FHN [15]. However, to date, the feasibility of automated segmentation has not been shown yet. This would improve the spatial assessment of necrotic lesions in addition to providing a more comprehensive disease staging. Ideally, quantification of FHN from 3D models would even be based on standard 2D MRI sequences, which are universally available and performed in the routine diagnostic workup of FHN. Through integrating necrotic bone volume and surface areas to better predict which patients will benefit from reconstructive surgery for FHN, as opposed to those with too advanced necrosis, a more objective staging of FHN could be achieved. Thus, in our study, we sought to evaluate a deep-learning method to automatically quantify the necrotic bone in FHN.

Our aims were to: (1) manually reconstruct MRI-based 3D models of FHN to calculate necrotic volume and surface area to serve as a reference standard for the manual segmentations based on a 2D MRI sequence; (2) use the manual segmentations of a 2D MRI sequence for the training and testing of a neural network for automated reconstruction and quantification of FHN; and (3) compare the quantification of femoral head necrosis and Kerboul angle between early and advanced ARCO stages.

## 2. Materials and Methods

This was an IRB-approved retrospective study of 26 patients (mean age 30 years, 14 men) with FHN diagnosed in a tertiary orthopedic university hospital. Diagnosis of FHN was established in patients with a history of hip symptoms at clinical examination. All patients underwent biplanar radiographic imaging with supine AP pelvis views and cross table lateral view and subsequent MRI of the hip. FHN was graded according to the commonly recommended 2019 ARCO grading [12]: I (negative x-rays): two hips; II (no fracture): four hips; IIIA (head collapse < 2 mm): 13 hips; IIIB (head collapse > 2 mm): 11 hips.

Patients underwent preoperative MR arthrography at 3T (Skyra, Siemens Healthineers, Erlangen, Germany) for their hips including the application of traction according to a previously described technique [16,17]. This included the acquisition of multiplanar proton-density (PD) weighted turbo spin-echo (TSE) imaging without fat saturation (coronal, radial and axial orientation) and a high-resolution axial-oblique 3D T1-weighted volume interpolated breath-hold examination (VIBE) sequence [18]. Sequence parameters for the coronal PD-w sequence were repetition time (TR)/echo time (TE), 2600/11 milliseconds (ms), slice thickness of 2 millimeters (mm), 170 × 170 mm field of view, matrix size of 269 × 384, acquisition time (AT) of 3 min. Sequence parameters for the 3D T1-w VIBE sequence were TR/TE, 15/3.3 ms, slice thickness of 0.8 mm, 160 × 160 mm field of view, matrix size of 192 × 192, and an acquisition time of 8:46 min.

Modified Kerboul angles were measured for each of the patients from the MR images, according to the method of Ha et al., where the greatest extension was assessed in the midcoronal and midsagittal planes and summed, since measuring from only the coronal plane is not as accurate in the quantification of necrosis [19]. Additionally, Tönnis scores to assess the degree of hip osteoarthritis were included, with grades from 0 (no osteoarthritis present) to 3 (large cysts, avascular necrosis, and severe narrowing of joint space) [20,21] (Table 1).

Table 1. Demography and radiography of the study population.

| Parameter | Mean ± SD/Number of Hips (%) |
|---|---|
| Patients (hips) | 26 (30 hips) |
| Age (Mean ± SD) | 30 ± 7 |
| Sex (male in%) | 53.85 |
| Etiology, hips | |
| Idiopathic (%) | 13 (43) |
| Posttraumatic (%) | 3 (10) |
| Systemic (%) | 11 (37) |
| Perthes Disease (%) | 3 (10) |
| Treatment, hips (%) | |
| Non-Operative Treatment | 12 (40) |
| Hip Arthroscopy | 0 (0) |
| Surgical Hip Dislocation (total) | 14 (47) |
| Concomitant Femoral Osteotomy | 5 (16) |
| Periacetabular Osteotomy | 1 * (3) |
| First Surgery: Total Arthroplasty | 3 (10) |
| Tönnis grade of osteoarthritis, hips (%) | |
| Tönnis grade < 2 | 28 (93) |
| Tönnis grade ≥ 2 | 2 (7) |
| ARCO grading | |
| ARCO I (%) | 2 (7) |
| ARCO II (%) | 4 (13) |
| ARCO IIIA (%) | 13 (43) |
| ARCO IIIB (%) | 11 (37) |
| Modified Kerboul angle (Mean ± SD°) | 198 ± 77 |

Values are expressed as the Mean ± Standard Deviation or as the number of hips and the percentage of the total; ARCO – Association Research Circulation Osseous Staging for osteonecrosis of the femoral head, * – surgical hip dislocation was also performed for this hip.

## 2.1. Manual and Automatic Segmentation of FHN

Manual segmentation of the necrotic bone and unaffected femoral head was performed by an expert reader on 3D T1 VIBE MRI and the coronal 2D PD-w sequence using Amira software (FEI; Hillsboro, Oregon, USA). The manual segmentations were then used to train a set of convolutional neural networks (nnU-Net) [22] (Figures 1 and 2). The neuronal network was tested with a 5-fold cross-validation scheme on the unseen data. The 5-fold cross-validation trains five different networks where 4/5 of the data are used to train and the remaining 1/5 to test the network. This has the advantage that the overall set can be used as unseen data in this configuration. Therefore, the ensemble of the five different networks built in the nnU-Net framework was not used. The architecture tested consisted of an ensembled 2D-3D U-Net that was applied on the coronal 2D PD-w TSE sequence. For the supervised deep learning approach, the manually segmented images were used as the ground truth, and the mean Dice coefficient was calculated.

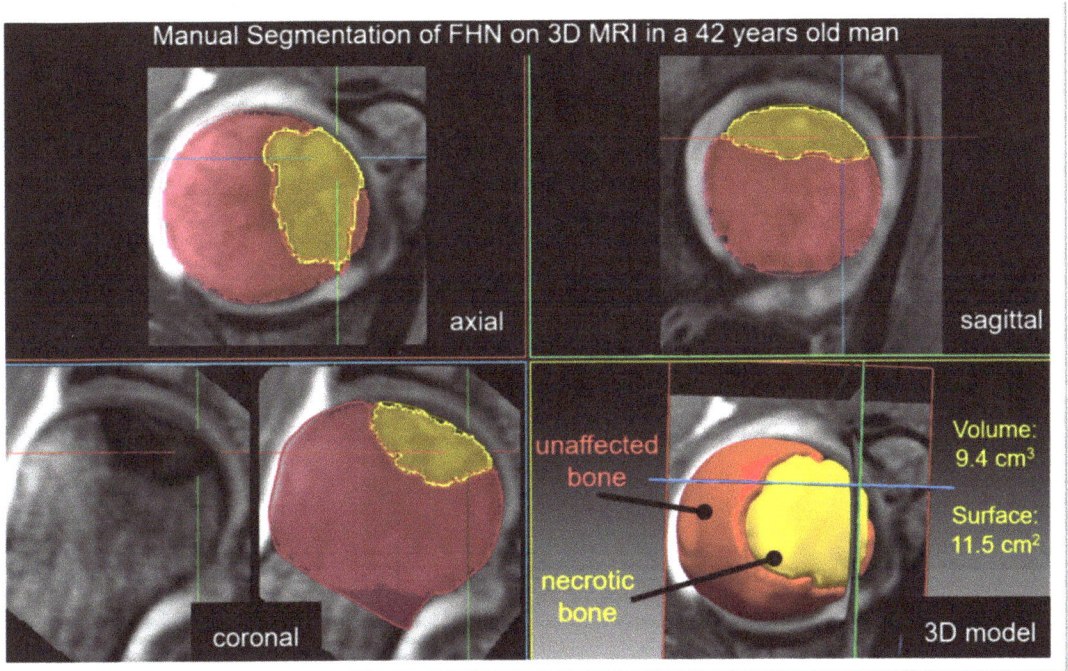

**Figure 1.** Manual segmentation of femoral head necrosis based on the 3D T1 volume interpolated breath-hold examination (VIBE) sequence is shown. The 3D sequence allows for multiplanar reformation for the threshold assisted 3D segmentation of the unaffected bone (red) and the necrotic bone (yellow). In this patient, this yielded a necrotic volume of 9.4 cm$^3$ and surface area of 11.5 cm$^2$.

Images were volume-cropped with a spacing of 160 × 30 × 160 voxels and 0.44 × 2.4 × 0.44 mm.

The network was trained for 60 epochs. Otherwise, the default settings were kept.

The volume and surface of the necrotic and unaffected region were calculated for the manual and the automatic segmentations from the neural network. The percent of necrotic bone volume and necrotic femoral head surface were calculated.

To calculate the surface, the segmentation was converted into a contour, and a plane was fitted to the flat portion where the segmentation ends in the femoral neck. Everything within a distance of 3 mm to the plane was removed and was not part of the surface of the femoral head. Then, the surface was calculated for the overall femoral head and the necrotic part.

### 2.2. Statistical Analysis

Dice coefficients were calculated to assess the accuracy of the automatic segmentation. The mean difference between the two manual segmentations plus the difference between the 2D manual segmentation and the automatic ones were compared with the paired *t*-tests and the correlation was assessed with the Pearson correlation coefficients. We then compared the absolute and relative size of the necrosis between early and advanced stages of AVN (ARCO I/II versus IIIA/B) using Mann–Whitney U tests. A *p*-value less than 0.05 determined the statistical significance. Pearson correlations were also run for the six parameters for each segmentation relative to the modified Kerboul angle.

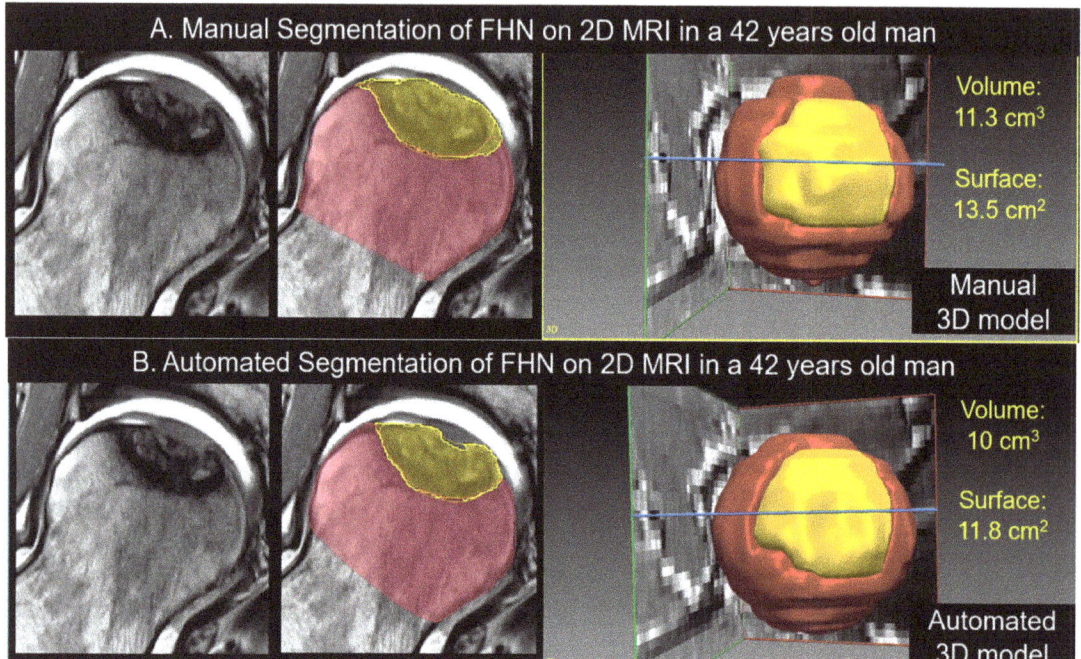

**Figure 2.** (**A**) Manual and (**B**) automatic segmentation of femoral head necrosis based on the 2D PD-w TSE sequence of the same patient as in Figure 1 is shown. Unaffected (red) and necrotic bone (yellow) were masked using threshold assisted (**A**) manual segmentation, which was used as the ground truth to train the neuronal network for (**B**) fully automatic segmentation. Automatic segmentation yielded comparable values as manual segmentation for relative necrotic volume (10 cm$^3$ vs. 11.3 cm$^3$) and relative necrotic surface area (11.8 cm$^2$ vs. 13.5 cm$^2$). Dice coefficient for necrotic bone was 90% and 94% for the unaffected bone.

## 3. Results

### 3.1. Manual Segmentation of 3D MRI versus Manual Segmentation of 2D MRI

Upon direct comparison, the ground truth manual segmentation of 3D MRI was consistent with the manual segmentation of 2D MRI. The mean differences and 95% confidence intervals (CI) between the 3D and 2D segmentations were $0.08 \pm 2.8$ cm$^3$ and $-0.97$ to 1.1 cm$^3$ (volume of necrosis), $1 \pm 6\%$ and $-2$ to 3% (percent of necrotic bone volume), $0.4 \pm 3.3$ cm$^2$ and $-0.9$ to 1.6 cm$^2$ (surface of necrotic bone), $-0.5 \pm 4.2$ cm$^2$ and $-2.1$ to 1.1 cm$^2$ (unaffected femoral surface), and $1 \pm 5\%$ and 1 to 3% (percent of necrotic femoral head surface). Each of these five parameters had *p*-values above the 0.05 threshold, except for the sixth parameter (volume of unaffected bone), which had a mean difference ($p = 0.0234$) and CI of $-1.5 \pm 3.4$ cm$^3$ and $-2.7$ to $-0.2$ cm$^3$, respectively. Furthermore, the correlations between the 3D and 2D segmentations for all six parameters were strong ($R_p > 0.9$), with $p < 0.001$ (Tables 2 and 3).

### 3.2. Manual Segmentation of 2D MRI Versus Automatic Segmentation of 2D MRI

Accuracy of the automatic segmentation as assessed with Dice coefficients for the automatic model were $75 \pm 15\%$ and $91 \pm 5\%$ for the necrotic and unaffected bone, respectively.

Upon direct comparison, the manual segmentation of 2D MRI was comparable with the automatic segmentation of 2D MRI (all $p > 0.05$). The mean differences and confidence intervals (CI) between the segmentations were $0.9 \pm 2.7$ cm$^3$ and $-0.1$ to $1.9$ cm$^3$ (volume of necrosis), $-0.8 \pm 2.8$ cm$^3$ and $-1.8$ to $0.3$ cm$^3$ (volume of unaffected bone), $2 \pm 5\%$ and $0$ to $4\%$ (percent of necrotic bone volume), $1.5 \pm 4$ cm$^2$ and $-0.01$ to $3$ cm$^2$ (surface of necrotic bone), $0.7 \pm 2.6$ cm$^2$ and $-0.3$ to $1.6$ cm$^2$ (unaffected femoral surface), and $3 \pm 7\%$ and $0$ to $5\%$ (percent of necrotic femoral head surface). Each of these six parameters showed strong correlations between the segmentations ($R_p > 0.9$), with $p < 0.001$ (Tables 2 and 4).

**Table 2.** Quantification of femoral head necrosis based on manual segmentations of 3D and 2D MRI and the automatic segmentation of 2D MRI using deep learning.

| Parameter | Manual Segmentation of 3D MRI | | Manual Segmentation of 2D MRI | | Automatic Segmentation of 2D MRI | |
| --- | --- | --- | --- | --- | --- | --- |
| | Mean ± SD | Range | Mean ± SD | Range | Mean ± SD | Range |
| Volume of necrosis (cm$^3$) | 8.9 ± 7.4 | 0.7 to 29 | 8.8 ± 7.4 | 0.6 to 28 | 7.9 ± 6.3 | 0.9 to 23 |
| Volume of unaffected bone (cm$^3$) | 39 ± 15 | 20 to 72 | 41 ± 15 | 20 to 71 | 42 ± 14 | 22 to 73 |
| Percent of necrotic bone volume (%) | 19 ± 15 | 2 to 59 | 18 ± 15 | 1 to 54 | 16 ± 13 | 2 to 47 |
| Surface of necrotic bone (cm$^2$) | 14 ± 9.3 | 1.3 to 35 | 13 ± 9.5 | 1.6 to 38 | 12 ± 8.2 | 0.8 to 33 |
| Unaffected femoral head surface (cm$^2$) | 59 ± 14 | 36 to 90 | 59 ± 13 | 42 to 87 | 59 ± 12 | 44 to 84 |
| Percent of necrotic femoral head surface (%) | 23 ± 15 | 2 to 58 | 23 ± 16 | 3 to 60 | 20 ± 14 | 2 to 54 |

Values are expressed as Mean ± Standard Deviation; cm = centimeters.

**Table 3.** Comparison of the manual segmentation of femoral head necrosis on 3D MRI with the manual segmentation of 2D MRI.

| Parameter | Difference (Mean ± SD) | CI | p Value | Correlation | p Value |
| --- | --- | --- | --- | --- | --- |
| Volume of necrosis (cm$^3$) | 0.08 ± 2.8 | −0.97 to 1.1 | 0.873 | $R_p = 0.928$ | <0.001 |
| Volume of unaffected bone (cm$^3$) | −1.5 ± 3.4 | −2.7 to −0.2 | 0.0234 | $R_p = 0.975$ | <0.001 |
| Percent of necrotic bone volume (%) | 1 ± 6 | −2 to 3 | 0.526 | $R_p = 0.928$ | <0.001 |
| Surface of necrotic bone (cm$^2$) | 0.4 ± 3.3 | −0.9 to 1.6 | 0.536 | $R_p = 0.938$ | <0.001 |
| Unaffected femoral head surface (cm$^2$) | −0.5 ± 4.2 | −2.1 to 1.1 | 0.515 | $R_p = 0.958$ | <0.001 |
| Percent of necrotic femoral head surface (%) | 1 ± 5 | 1 to 3 | 0.467 | $R_p = 0.940$ | <0.001 |

Difference values are expressed as Mean ± Standard Deviation; CI are the 95% confidence intervals; $R_p$ denotes the Pearson correlation coefficient.

**Table 4.** Comparison of manual versus automatic segmentation of FHN based on 2D MRI.

| Parameter | Difference, Mean ± SD | CI | p Value | Correlation | p Value |
| --- | --- | --- | --- | --- | --- |
| Volume of necrosis (cm$^3$) | 0.9 ± 2.7 | −0.1 to 1.9 | 0.0858 | $R_p = 0.936$ | <0.001 |
| Volume of unaffected bone (cm$^3$) | −0.8 ± 2.8 | −1.8 to 0.3 | 0.152 | $R_p = 0.982$ | <0.001 |
| Percent of necrotic bone volume (%) | 2 ± 5 | 0 to 4 | 0.10 | $R_p = 0.935$ | <0.001 |
| Necrotic bone surface (cm$^2$) | 1.5 ± 4 | −0.01 to 3 | 0.0517 | $R_p = 0.910$ | <0.001 |
| Unaffected femoral head surface (cm$^2$) | 0.7 ± 2.6 | −0.3 to 1.6 | 0.173 | $R_p = 0.979$ | <0.001 |
| Percent of necrotic femoral head surface (%) | 3 ± 7 | 0 to 5 | 0.0641 | $R_p = 0.892$ | <0.001 |

Difference values are expressed as Mean ± Standard Deviation; CI are the 95% confidence intervals; $R_p$ denotes the Pearson correlation coefficient.

### 3.3. Quantitative Comparison of Early and Advanced Stages of Femoral Head Necrosis

No significant difference ($p = 0.0775$) was observed for the modified Kerboul angle between hips with early versus advanced FHN (median of 153°, interquartile range of 58° versus 195°, 70°) (Table 5).

For the manual 2D segmentation, examination of the six aforementioned parameters between early (ARCO 0-II) and advanced (ARCO > II) FHN demonstrated significant differences (all $p < 0.05$) for volume of necrosis, percent of necrotic bone volume, necrotic bone surface, and percent of necrotic femoral head surface. Accordingly, the median and (interquartile ranges) reported for these parameters between early and advanced stages were 2.2 (2.7) vs. 8.9 (10.1), 4 (8) vs. 15 (16), 4.5 (4) vs. 12 (13.6), and 8 (10) vs. 20 (26) (Table 5).

Table 5. Comparison of the manual and automatic segmentation of femoral head necrosis based on 2D MRI between hips with early versus advanced disease stages.

| Parameters | Manual 2D Segmentation Median (IQR) | | | Automatic 2D Segmentation Median (IQR) | | |
|---|---|---|---|---|---|---|
| | ARCO 0-II | ARCO > II | p-Value | ARCO 0-II | ARCO > II | p-Value |
| Modified Kerboul angle (°) | 153 (58) | 195 (70) | 0.0775 | 153 (58) | 195 (70) | 0.0775 |
| Volume of necrosis (cm$^3$) | 2.2 (2.7) | 8.9 (10.1) | 0.0133 | 2.2 (4) | 8.8 (7.9) | 0.0257 |
| Volume of unaffected bone (cm$^3$) | 40 (12.2) | 36 (19.2) | 0.315 | 41 (9.9) | 37 (12.5) | 0.270 |
| Percent of necrotic bone volume (%) | 4 (8) | 15 (16) | 0.0226 | 6 (6) | 13 (16) | 0.0199 |
| Necrotic bone surface (cm$^2$) | 4.5 (4) | 12 (13.6) | 0.0152 | 4.8 (3.6) | 12 (8.2) | 0.0133 |
| Unaffected femoral head surface (cm$^2$) | 54 (12) | 55 (16) | 0.713 | 52 (12) | 55 (16) | 0.825 |
| Percent of necrotic femoral head surface (%) | 8 (10) | 20 (26) | 0.0257 | 9 (4) | 21 (12) | 0.0116 |

IQR = interquartile range; ARCO (Association Research Circulation Osseous Staging) where >2 indicates an advanced stage of femoral necrosis.

Automatic 2D segmentation analysis followed the pattern of the manual 2D segmentation, in which significant differences ($p < 0.05$) were found for the volume of necrosis, percent of necrotic bone volume, necrotic bone surface, and percent of necrotic femoral head surface between early and advanced stages of FHN. The median and (interquartile ranges) reported for these parameters between the early and advanced stages were 2.2 (4) vs. 8.8 (7.9), 6 (6) vs. 13 (16), 4.8 (3.6) vs. 12 (8.2), and 9 (4) vs. 21 (12) (Table 5).

Additional correlation with the modified Kerboul angle was assessed for each of the three segmentations (manual 3D, manual 2D, and automatic 2D) across the four parameters of necrosis quantification. Strong correlations were present ($R_p > 0.85$) for the volume of necrosis, percent of necrotic bone, surface of necrotic bone, and percent of necrotic femoral head surface, with all correlations being significant ($p < 0.001$) (Table 6). Despite these high correlations between modified Kerboul angles and 3D quantification of FHN, we observed marked differences in the relative necrotic volume and relative necrotic surface area in some patients with comparable Kerboul angles (Figure 3).

Table 6. Correlations between the manual segmentation of 3D and 2D MRI and automatic segmentation of 2D MRI against the modified Kerboul angle.

| Parameter | Manual Segmentation of 3D MRI | | Manual Segmentation of 2D MRI | | Automatic Segmentation of 2D MRI | |
|---|---|---|---|---|---|---|
| | vs Modified Kerboul | p-Value | vs Modified Kerboul | p-Value | vs Modified Kerboul | p-Value |
| Volume of necrosis (cm$^3$) | $R_p = 0.859$ | <0.001 | $R_p = 0.865$ | <0.001 | $R_p = 0.867$ | <0.001 |
| Percent of necrotic bone volume (%) | $R_p = 0.883$ | <0.001 | $R_p = 0.896$ | <0.001 | $R_p = 0.913$ | <0.001 |
| Surface of necrotic bone (cm$^2$) | $R_p = 0.861$ | <0.001 | $R_p = 0.869$ | <0.001 | $R_p = 0.866$ | <0.001 |
| Percent of necrotic femoral head surface (%) | $R_p = 0.881$ | <0.001 | $R_p = 0.881$ | <0.001 | $R_p = 0.909$ | <0.001 |

$R_p$ denotes the Pearson correlation coefficient.

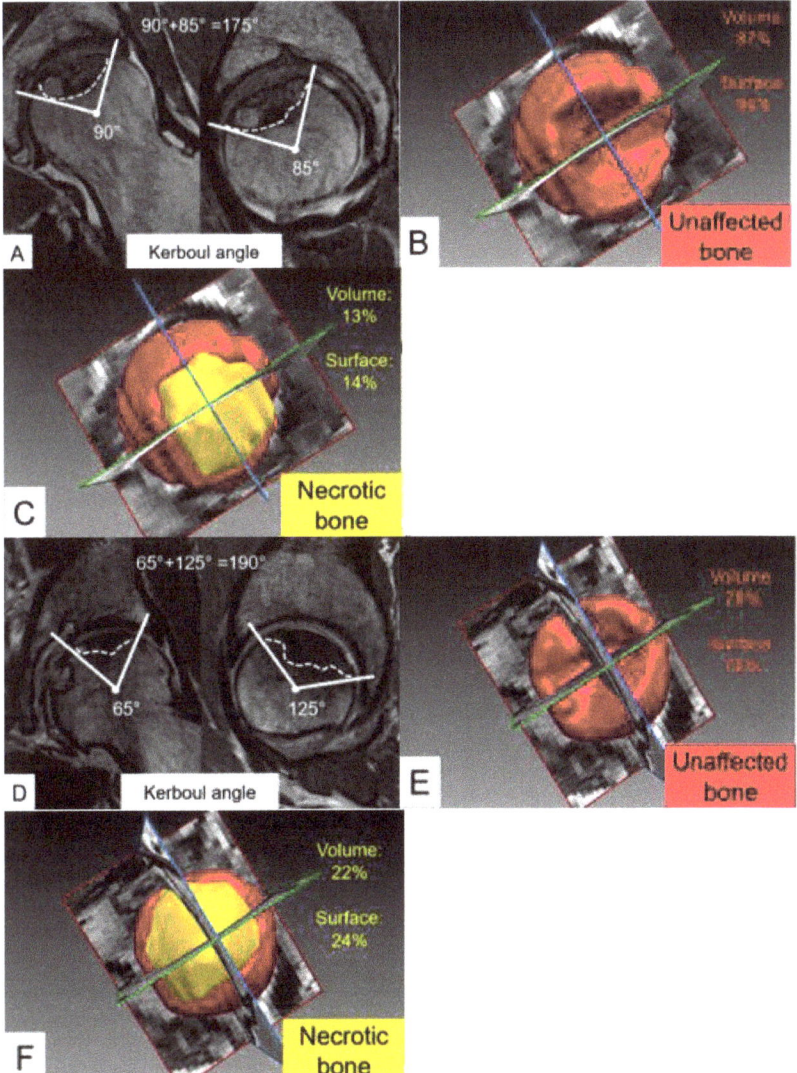

**Figure 3.** Quantification of femoral head necrosis with modified Kerboul angles and 3D quantification using fully automated 3D models of the femoral head in two different patients. (**A–C**) 43-year-old man and (**C–F**) 36-year-old woman with advanced femoral head necrosis (ARCO 3A) and comparable Kerboul angles of (**A**) 175° and (**D**) 190°. In contrast, marked differences were observed between both patients for (**C,F**) relative necrotic volume (13% versus 22%) and relative necrotic surface area (14% versus 24%), underlining the potential of deep learning-based 3D quantification to improve surgical planning.

## 4. Discussion

In its progression, FHN leads to the collapse of the femoral head in a large number of patients, with 67% developing collapse even without the manifestation of clinical symptoms [12,23]. Accurate disease staging is thus imperative for FHN to dictate the right course of treatment, particularly in younger patients who may be able to avoid total hip arthroplasty and preserve the native joint [24]. Within our work, we sought to expand upon the current FHN staging and Kerboul angle through the inclusion of 3D volumetric and surface area quantification of necrotic lesions. We retrospectively analyzed the MRIs of 26 patients (30 hips) with FHN and varying ARCO stages upon which we performed the manual segmentation of FHN based on a 3D T1-w sequence. The segmentation of the 3D sequence served as the reference standard as it has high-spatial resolution with thin and continuous slices alike. Since numerous different 3D MRI sequences are available and not routinely performed in the workup for FHN, we further compared segmentation accuracy using the standard 2D PD-w TSE sequence and subsequent automatic segmentation using a supervised deep learning approach. Indeed, we could show that accurate quantification of FHN was possible when performed manually and fully automatically on 2D MRI (Tables 2–4). To the best of our knowledge, our study is the first to show that deep learning based segmentation is accurate for the 3D quantification of femoral head necrosis. Previous studies were successful in being comparable to orthopedic surgeons in diagnosing necrosis [25–27], with one study in particular utilizing 3D MRIs to allow for a potentially earlier diagnosis of femoral necrosis [25]. Our study also demonstrated this, as we found it to be equivalent across the six parameters of necrosis (Table 4) and correlates equally well with the modified Kerboul angle as the other manual segmentations (Table 6). This shows that not only was the automatic model accurate, but volumetric parameters (such as volume of necrosis and percent of necrotic bone) and surface ones (surface of necrotic bone and percent of necrotic femoral head surface) could be just as viable to predict necrosis as the modified Kerboul angle parameter.

Kerboul angle, as first described by Kerboul et al. [28], is a method to evaluate the total necrotic angle from lateral and anterior-posterior radiographs, which was then improved upon with the advent of the MRI [29]. The modified Kerboul angle is now typically used to assess the extent of necrosis to predict future collapse, being the sum of the necrotic angles in the coronal and sagittal planes on the MRI, and has shown promise [30]. However, as Steinberg et al. pointed out in their study, the modified Kerboul angle is more variable than parameters such as the index of necrosis and the modified index of necrosis, even when assuming a percentage of femoral head involvement from a 250-degree angle for the head rather than the 180-degree angle, which was previously implemented [31,32]. Our results seem to support the notion that the modified Kerboul angle is a less sensitive metric relative to the 3D volumetric assessment, given that the volume of necrosis, percent of necrotic bone volume, necrotic bone surface, and percent of necrotic femoral head were all significantly different between early and advanced staged ARCO whereas the Kerboul angle was not (Table 5). Although our sample size was not sufficient to perform subgroup analysis between hips with focal or more extensive FHN, we could observe marked differences when performing automated quantification of FHN compared to measuring the Kerboul angles alone (Figure 3). Other studies have also demonstrated the difficulty in measuring the actual size of a 3D lesion with 2D angular measurements [31,33,34].

Currently, the ARCO classification is widely utilized to distinguish between the different stages of AVN based on MRI, radiograph, and the degree of femoral depression in the more advanced stages [12]. However, 3D volumetric assessment was not incorporated in this analysis to better categorize the stages, which could prove invaluable in ensuring that patients undergo the essential surgical course [35]. Based on our results, the quantification for volume and surface area were more sensitive than the Kerboul angle, and should be used to make ARCO staging and AVN diagnosis more robust clinically. Furthermore, our results confirm that the amount of necrosis in terms of volume and surface area increased from the threshold of ARCO stage II, indicating that once collapse takes place, there is indeed a substantial change in the joint (Table 5) [36].

Our study had some limitations, the most significant being that all of the patient scans were acquired with the same site and same MRI vendor. As has been pointed out in previous deep learning studies, sufficient training of these models requires scans from multiple MR machines and sites to improve generalizability [37,38]. Our study paves the way for future work implementing this approach at multiple sites with scanners from different vendors, as we have demonstrated that our automatic segmentation could perform equally well to our ground truth segmentations in the quantification of FHN. Another limitation is our sample size, which although somewhat smaller due to the lower prevalence of disease, should be expanded in follow-up studies to both improve the performance of the model and ensure there is no overfitting or undertraining [36]. Finally, our study was retrospective in nature, leading to potential selection bias with the number of hips included that were in the advanced ARCO stage (IIIA or IIIB) relative to the early stages (ARCO I and II). This could have skewed some of the values obtained for the six parameters for the manual segmentations and the automatic model.

In conclusion, our deep learning model for AVN proved to be just as accurate as our ground truth and is the first to accurately quantify necrosis based on 3D models of the femur. Such models could be further used for 3D printing or finite element analysis to better simulate the effect of different surgical approaches for treatment of the necrotic lesion. Furthermore, we were able to corroborate the findings of previous studies that the modified Kerboul angle is not the most sensitive metric, and proposed/identified four parameters that outperformed it when distinguishing between early and advanced necrosis. While larger and more heterogeneous studies need to be carried out as well as continued improvement of AVN staging, this study will hopefully allow for further work to optimize surgical decision making and ameliorate patient outcomes with the disease in the near future.

**Author Contributions:** Conceptualization, A.C.R., A.K.N. and F.S.; Methodology, A.C.R., A.K.N., M.K.M., T.D.L., S.D.S., S.V., A.B., M.T., K.A.S., N.G. and F.S.; Software, A.C.R., A.K.N., S.V., A.B., N.V., N.G. and F.S.; Validation, A.C.R., A.K.N., M.K.M., T.D.L., S.V., A.B., N.G. and F.S.; Formal analysis, A.C.R., A.K.N., S.V., A.B., N.V., N.G. and F.S.; Investigation, A.C.R., A.K.N., S.V., A.B., M.T. and F.S.; Resources, S.D.S., M.T., K.A.S., N.G. and F.S.; Data curation, A.C.R., A.K.N., S.V., A.B., N.G. and F.S.; Writing—original draft preparation, A.C.R., A.K.N., M.K.M., T.D.L., S.D.S., S.V., A.B., N.V., M.T., K.A.S., N.G. and F.S.; Writing—review and editing, A.C.R., A.K.N., M.K.M., T.D.L., S.D.S., S.V., A.B., N.V., M.T., K.A.S., N.G. and F.S.; Visualization, A.C.R., A.K.N. and F.S.; Supervision, S.D.S., M.T., K.A.S., N.G. and F.S.; Project administration, S.D.S., M.T., K.A.S., N.G. and F.S.; Funding acquisition, F.S. All authors have read and agreed to the published version of the manuscript.

**Funding:** This study was funded by the Swiss National Science Foundation (Grant Number 205091) and the clinical trial unit of the University of Bern.

**Institutional Review Board Statement:** The study was conducted in accordance with the Declaration of Helsinki, and approved by the Institutional Review Board (or Ethics Committee) of the University of Bern (protocol code 2018-00078, date of approval 13 February 2018).

**Informed Consent Statement:** Patient consent was waived due to the retrospective nature of the study.

**Data Availability Statement:** As per the national guidelines, sharing of data was not applicable.

**Conflicts of Interest:** The funders had no role in the design of the study; in the collection, analyses, or interpretation of data; in the writing of the manuscript; or in the decision to publish the results.

## References

1. Bassounas, A.E.; Karantanas, A.H.; Fotiadis, D.I.; Malizos, K.N. Femoral head osteonecrosis: Volumetric MRI assessment and outcome. *Eur. J. Radiol.* **2007**, *63*, 10–15. [CrossRef] [PubMed]
2. Banerjee, S.; Kapadia, B.H.; Jauregui, J.J.; Cherian, J.J.; Mont, M.A. Natural History of Osteonecrosis. In *Osteonecrosis*; Koo, K.H., Mont, M., Jones, L., Eds.; Springer: Berlin/Heidelberg, Germany, 2014; pp. 161–164. [CrossRef]
3. Mont, M.A.; Salem, H.S.; Piuzzi, N.S.; Goodman, S.B.; Jones, L.C. Nontraumatic Osteonecrosis of the Femoral Head: Where Do We Stand Today? A 5-Year Update. *J. Bone Jt. Surg.* **2020**, *102*, 1084–1099. [CrossRef]
4. Lubega, N.; Mkandawire, N.C.; Sibande, G.C.; Norrish, A.R.; Harrison, W.J. Joint replacement in Malawi. *J. Bone Jt. Surg.* **2009**, *91*, 341–343. [CrossRef]
5. Steppacher, S.D.; Sedlmayer, R.; Tannast, M.; Schmaranzer, F.; A Siebenrock, K. Surgical hip dislocation with femoral osteotomy and bone grafting prevents head collapse in hips with advanced necrosis. *HIP Int. J. Clin. Exp. Res. Hip Pathol. Ther.* **2019**, *30*, 398–406. [CrossRef]

6. Chughtai, M.; Piuzzi, N.S.; Khlopas, A.; Jones, L.C.; Goodman, S.B.; Mont, M.A. An evidence-based guide to the treatment of osteonecrosis of the femoral head. *Bone Jt. J.* **2017**, *99-B*, 1267–1279. [CrossRef] [PubMed]
7. McAuley, J.P.; Szuszczewicz, E.S.; Young, A.; A Engh, C. Total Hip Arthroplasty in Patients 50 Years and Younger. *Clin. Orthop. Relat. Res.* **2004**, *418*, 119–125. [CrossRef] [PubMed]
8. Cao, L.; Guo, C.; Chen, J.; Chen, Z.; Yan, Z. Free Vascularized Fibular Grafting Improves Vascularity Compared with Core Decompression in Femoral Head Osteonecrosis: A Randomized Clinical Trial. *Clin. Orthop. Relat. Res.* **2017**, *475*, 2230–2240. [CrossRef]
9. Camp, J.F.; Colwell, C.W. Core decompression of the femoral head for osteonecrosis. *J. Bone Jt. Surg.* **1986**, *68*, 1313–1319. [CrossRef]
10. Sugioka, Y.; Yamamoto, T. Transtrochanteric Posterior Rotational Osteotomy for Osteonecrosis. *Clin. Orthop. Relat. Res.* **2008**, *466*, 1104–1109. [CrossRef]
11. Ganz, R.; Gill, T.J.; Gautier, E.; Ganz, K.; Krügel, N.; Berlemann, U. Surgical dislocation of the adult hip. *J. Bone Jt. Surg.* **2001**, *83*, 1119–1124. [CrossRef]
12. Yoon, B.-H.; Mont, M.A.; Koo, K.-H.; Chen, C.-H.; Cheng, E.Y.; Cui, Q.; Drescher, W.; Gangji, V.; Goodman, S.B.; Ha, Y.-C.; et al. The 2019 Revised Version of Association Research Circulation Osseous Staging System of Osteonecrosis of the Femoral Head. *J. Arthroplast.* **2019**, *35*, 933–940. [CrossRef] [PubMed]
13. Karantanas, A.H.; E Drakonaki, E. The Role of MR Imaging in Avascular Necrosis of the Femoral Head. *Semin. Musculoskelet. Radiol.* **2011**, *15*, 281–300. [CrossRef] [PubMed]
14. Cherian, S.F.; Laorr, A.; Saleh, K.J.; Kuskowski, M.A.; Bailey, R.F.; Cheng, E.Y. Quantifying the extent of femoral head involvement in osteonecrosis. *J. Bone Jt. Surg.* **2003**, *85*, 309–315. [CrossRef] [PubMed]
15. Schmaranzer, F.; Todorski, I.A.S.; Lerch, T.D.; Schwab, J.; Cullmann-Bastian, J.; Tannast, M. Intra-articular Lesions: Imaging and Surgical Correlation. *Semin. Musculoskelet. Radiol.* **2017**, *21*, 487–506. [CrossRef]
16. Meier, M.K.; Lerch, T.D.; Steppacher, S.D.; Siebenrock, K.A.; Tannast, M.; Vavron, P.; Schmaranzer, E.; Schmaranzer, F. High prevalence of hip lesions secondary to arthroscopic over- or undercorrection of femoroacetabular impingement in patients with postoperative pain. *Eur. Radiol.* **2021**, *32*, 3097–3111. [CrossRef]
17. Schmaranzer, F.; Lerch, T.D.; Steppacher, S.D.; A Siebenrock, K.; Tannast, M. Femoral cartilage damage occurs at the zone of femoral head necrosis and can be accurately detected on traction MR arthrography of the hip in patients undergoing joint preserving hip surgery. *J. Hip Preserv. Surg.* **2021**, *8*, 28–39. [CrossRef]
18. Schmaranzer, F.; Helfenstein, R.; Zeng, G.; Lerch, T.; Novais, E.N.; Wylie, J.D.; Kim, Y.-J.; Siebenrock, K.A.; Tannast, M.; Zheng, G. Automatic MRI-Based Three-Dimensional Models of Hip Cartilage Provide Improved Morphologic and Biochemical Analysis. *Clin. Orthop. Relat. Res.* **2019**, *477*, 1036–1052. [CrossRef]
19. Ha, Y.-C.; Jung, W.H.; Kim, J.-R.; Seong, N.H.; Kim, S.-Y.; Koo, K.-H. Prediction of Collapse in Femoral Head Osteonecrosis: A Modified Kerboul Method with Use of Magnetic Resonance Images. *J. Bone Jt. Surg.* **2006**, *88*, 35–40. [CrossRef]
20. Tönnis, D.; Heinecke, A. Current Concepts Review—Acetabular and Femoral Anteversion. *J. Bone Jt. Surg.* **1999**, *81*, 1747–1770. [CrossRef]
21. Kovalenko, B.; Bremjit, P.; Fernando, N. Classifications in Brief: Tönnis Classification of Hip Osteoarthritis. *Clin. Orthop. Relat. Res.* **2018**, *476*, 1680–1684. [CrossRef]
22. Isensee, F.; Jaeger, P.F.; Kohl, S.A.A.; Petersen, J.; Maier-Hein, K.H. nnU-Net: A self-configuring method for deep learning-based biomedical image segmentation. *Nat. Methods* **2020**, *18*, 203–211. [CrossRef] [PubMed]
23. Tan, Y.; He, H.; Wan, Z.; Qin, J.; Wen, Y.; Pan, Z.; Wang, H.; Chen, L. Study on the outcome of patients with aseptic femoral head necrosis treated with percutaneous multiple small-diameter drilling core decompression: A retrospective cohort study based on magnetic resonance imaging and equivalent sphere model analysis. *J. Orthop. Surg. Res.* **2020**, *15*, 264. [CrossRef] [PubMed]
24. Arbab, D.; König, D.P. Atraumatic Femoral Head Necrosis in Adults. *Dtsch. Ärzteblatt Int.* **2016**, *113*, 31–38. [CrossRef] [PubMed]
25. Wang, P.; Liu, X.; Xu, J.; Li, T.; Sun, W.; Li, Z.; Gao, F.; Shi, L.; Li, Z.; Wu, X.; et al. Deep learning for diagnosing osteonecrosis of the femoral head based on magnetic resonance imaging. *Comput. Methods Programs Biomed.* **2021**, *208*, 106229. [CrossRef]
26. Zhu, L.; Han, J.; Guo, R.; Wu, D.; Wei, Q.; Chai, W.; Tang, S. An Automatic Classification of the Early Osteonecrosis of Femoral Head with Deep Learning. *Curr. Med. Imaging* **2021**, *16*, 1323–1331. [CrossRef]
27. Li, Y.; Tian, H. Deep Learning-Based End-to-End Diagnosis System for Avascular Necrosis of Femoral Head. *IEEE J. Biomed. Health Inform.* **2020**, *25*, 2093–2102. [CrossRef]
28. Kerboul, M.; Thomine, J.; Postel, M.; Merle d'Aubigné, R. The conservative surgical treatment of idiopathic aseptic necrosis of the femoral head. *J. Bone Jt. Surg.* **1974**, *56*, 291–296. [CrossRef]
29. Boontanapibul, K.; Huddleston, J.I.; Amanatullah, D.F.; Maloney, W.J.; Goodman, S.B. Modified Kerboul Angle Predicts Outcome of Core Decompression with or without Additional Cell Therapy. *J. Arthroplast.* **2021**, *36*, 1879–1886. [CrossRef]
30. Steinberg, M.E.; Oh, S.C.; Khoury, V.; Udupa, J.K.; Steinberg, D.R. Lesion size measurement in femoral head necrosis. *Int. Orthop.* **2018**, *42*, 1585–1591. [CrossRef]
31. Koo, K.H.; Kim, R. Quantifying the extent of osteonecrosis of the femoral head. A new method using MRI. *J. Bone Jt. Surg.* **1995**, *77*, 875–880. [CrossRef]
32. Theodorou, D.J.; Malizos, K.N.; Beris, A.E.; Theodorou, S.J.; Soucacos, P.N. Multimodal Imaging Quantitation of the Lesion Size in Osteonecrosis of the Femoral Head. *Clin. Orthop. Relat. Res.* **2001**, *386*, 54–63. [CrossRef]

33. Steinberg, D.R.; Steinberg, M.E.; Garino, J.P.; Dalinka, M.; Udupa, J.K. Determining Lesion Size in Osteonecrosis of the Femoral Head. *J. Bone Jt. Surg.* **2006**, *88*, 27–34. [CrossRef]
34. Beck, D.M.; Park, B.K.; Youm, T.; Wolfson, T.S. Arthroscopic Treatment of Labral Tears and Concurrent Avascular Necrosis of the Femoral Head in Young Adults. *Arthrosc. Tech.* **2013**, *2*, e367–e371. [CrossRef]
35. Vora, A. Management of osteonecrosis in children and young adults with acute lymphoblastic leukaemia. *Br. J. Haematol.* **2011**, *155*, 549–560. [CrossRef]
36. Klontzas, M.E.; Stathis, I.; Spanakis, K.; Zibis, A.H.; Marias, K.; Karantanas, A.H. Deep Learning for the Differential Diagnosis between Transient Osteoporosis and Avascular Necrosis of the Hip. *Diagnostics* **2022**, *12*, 1870. [CrossRef]
37. Bento, M.; Fantini, I.; Park, J.; Rittner, L.; Frayne, R. Deep Learning in Large and Multi-Site Structural Brain MR Imaging Datasets. *Front. Neuroinform.* **2022**, *15*, 805669. [CrossRef]
38. Gao, Y.; Xiao, X.; Han, B.; Li, G.; Ning, X.; Wang, D.; Cai, W.; Kikinis, R.; Berkovsky, S.; Di Ieva, A.; et al. Deep Learning Methodology for Differentiating Glioma Recurrence from Radiation Necrosis Using Multimodal Magnetic Resonance Imaging: Algorithm Development and Validation. *JMIR Med. Inform.* **2020**, *8*, e19805. [CrossRef]

**Disclaimer/Publisher's Note:** The statements, opinions and data contained in all publications are solely those of the individual author(s) and contributor(s) and not of MDPI and/or the editor(s). MDPI and/or the editor(s) disclaim responsibility for any injury to people or property resulting from any ideas, methods, instructions or products referred to in the content.

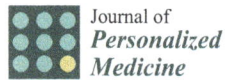

*Editorial*

# Cutting-Edge Approaches in Arthroplasty: Before, during and after Surgery

**Johannes Beckmann [1],\*, David Barrett [2] and Emmanuel Thienpont [3]**

1. Clinic for Orthopaedic and Trauma Surgery, Hospital Barmherzige Brüder Munich, 80639 München, Germany
2. Professor of Orthopaedic BioEngineering, School of Engineering Science, University of Southampton, Southampton SO17 1BJ, UK
3. Saint-Luc University Clinics, Department of Orthopedics and Musculoskeletal Traumatology, Catholic University of Louvain (UCLouvain), Avenue Hippocrate 10, 1200 Brussels, Belgium
* Correspondence: drjbeckmann@gmx.de

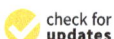

Citation: Beckmann, J.; Barrett, D.; Thienpont, E. Cutting-Edge Approaches in Arthroplasty: Before, during and after Surgery. *J. Pers. Med.* 2022, 12, 1671. https://doi.org/10.3390/jpm12101671

Received: 22 September 2022
Accepted: 29 September 2022
Published: 8 October 2022

**Publisher's Note:** MDPI stays neutral with regard to jurisdictional claims in published maps and institutional affiliations.

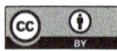

**Copyright:** © 2022 by the authors. Licensee MDPI, Basel, Switzerland. This article is an open access article distributed under the terms and conditions of the Creative Commons Attribution (CC BY) license (https://creativecommons.org/licenses/by/4.0/).

Personalised medicine was introduced in arthroplasty a long time ago with the aim of respecting each individual person for their unique personal characteristics in order to further improve outcomes. Compared to the early days of arthroplasty, the range of implant types, implant sizes, geometrical forms and implantation techniques has grown enormously in recent decades to deal better with the patients' needs and their anatomy. Some of those technical evolutions were lauded as being the new holy grail, but most disappeared again or were assembled within the existing technique as a small upgrade.

The developments in hip arthroplasty seem to be less radical and more conservative, because of the longevity of the implants and the high satisfaction rates of patients. In knee arthroplasty, 20% to 30% remain dissatisfied, urging surgeons, designers and implant companies to find solutions to their problems.

In the past two decades, sizing issues, such as overhang and pain or downsizing and flexion instability, have been addressed. This led to the development of many different sizes with more representative anatomical aspect ratios and better surface matching in almost all modern implants, and culminated in true customised implants manufactured on a per-patient basis [1–4].

There has also been a renaissance in partial knee replacements, where resurfacing of only the diseased side of the knee can lead to better results. This could be performed in possibly up to 50% of patients instead of using totals. The counterpoint of a threefold higher revision rate of partials compared to total knees can be clearly disarmed by surgical experience and, lately, also for the first time by registry data. The German arthroplasty registry (EPRD) shows a non-inferiority of revision rates in those clinics performing a high volume of partial knees [5–9].

The latest debate concerning individuality in knee arthroplasty is the debate and trend towards personalized alignment. Each human being has their own unique type of coronal alignment. The idea is to approach this native alignment more closely with an oblique implant position. To be able to obtain these more complex goals in surgery, new technologies are needed, with the newest trend certainly being precision-enabling robots. Paradoxically, all these precision-enabling techniques such as robots, computer navigation or patient-specific instruments were used for a decade to avoid surgical outliers outside of the neutral mechanical axis. Now, they help to implant the same prostheses in different outlier positions. This new trend clearly shows that the target for coronal alignment has changed. It only remains to be proven that this improves the subjective outcome of the patient and will not lead to reduced survivorship. The new generation of robots combines the advantages and precision of navigation and robotics. It is indisputable that precision is higher with the help of these technologies compared to conventional jigs and eye-balling, even compared to experienced surgeons. However, thorough planning is mandatory to avoid a possible "trash in—trash out" effect [10–17].

The difficulty with knee arthroplasty remains that all implants are made from metal and plastic and that they are supposed to substitute for cartilage, menisci and soft tissue structures such as ligaments. Furthermore, their shapes and radii of curvature were decided more than 40 years ago, mainly with the ambition of avoiding early failure of the materials. Today, these symmetrical implants ask for advanced technological tools to implant them asymmetrically into the native knee joint. Designing asymmetrical implants that respect the individual offsets of each part of the human knee might be a better evolution. Today, this remains difficult because of the logistics coming with this type of treatment and the high costs. However, if with the economy of scales and a higher volume of usage, the cost of goods can be reduced, this might be a more appealing concept for the future of arthroplasty. If this is combined with a robotic type of surgery, reducing the need for instrument sets and the patient-specific knee eliminates inventory, the value-chain of orthopaedics will have gone through its first new economic revolution in decades.

However, it is not only the "hardware" that makes the difference. The "software" of better peri-operative management of the patient has become a milestone in arthroplasty outcomes. Early mobilization, because of minimally invasive surgery, and improved pain and anaesthetic protocols are just some examples. Most of the dogmas that have existed in surgery for decades, and are transmitted from generation to generation of surgeons, were questioned and critically analysed. Postoperative drains were abandoned, the need for high pressure tourniquets was discussed and antifibrinolytic agents and local infiltration analgesia were introduced. The importance of clinical outcome for those changes are indisputable. While, a few decades ago, patients had to spend several weeks in hospital or even in bed following a joint replacement, arthroplasty has now become a procedure that is performed in outpatient surgery centres, where patients can leave the institution on the same day [18–22].

The growing importance of digitalization and collecting "big data" is relentless and one of the main topics for the future. The ultimate goal in arthroplasty will be to predict which technique and what system will help which patient with their unique anatomy. The collection of such "big data" physiologically and psychologically, pre-, intra- as well as postoperatively, together with expectations, satisfaction, capabilities and restrictions, will lead us to understand the real needs of our patients.

Although registers pool all arthroplasties performed, which initially does not seem to be very individual, national registers have to play a major role in documenting the quality of different implants and arthroplasty care overall, in order to describe best practice and report implant outliers. The registers have to be used for research and post-market surveillance, and register data may be a source for intelligent decision tools that can ultimately help to treat every individual patient better. This also helps in collecting "big data". Predictive tools based on machine-learning algorithms could reform clinical practice, especially when combining machine-learning algorithms with data from nationwide arthroplasty registries [23–32].

Furthermore, early detection and prevention of arthritic changes in the joint, resulting in the need for arthroplasty, are also changing and will continue to do so. Radiological detection becomes more subtle with reduced radiation exposure and fast and broad availability by digitalization. The understanding of pathology and early treatment options improves almost day by day. Concerning arthroplasty, tissue engineering is just one aspect. Given the enormous increase in the risks of bone and cartilage defects with the increase in aging population, the current treatments available are insufficient for handling this burden, and the supply of donor organs for transplantation is limited. Therefore, tissue engineering is a promising approach for treating such defects. Advances in materials research and high-tech optimized fabrication of scaffolds have increased the efficiency of tissue engineering [33–45].

Pharmacological innovation might become important for the prevention of osteoarthritis in the near future, too. Surgeons remember how rheumatoid arthritis patients were their main segment of arthroplasty patients because of severe joint destruction and important deformities. Since the introduction of disease-modifying drugs, that segment of patients has severely changed [35,46–48].

One big issue and remaining problem for the coming years and decades to come is the revision arthroplasty of failed implants. Even with optimized implantation and improved materials, the more active patients operated on today will potentially need new surgeries in the future. The threshold age for arthroplasty is also coming down in patients operated on for sports traumatology in the past and who are experiencing early osteoarthritis. More surgeries in the elderly population and multi-operated patients will potentially lead to more peri-prosthetic infections, requiring revision surgeries. Issues such as instability and aseptic loosening often need to be addressed within the first years after the index procedure. The removal of implants, infection and osteolysis can lead to bone loss and the need for bone substitution with cones or resection-type implants. The number of implanted megaprostheses grows exponentially, as does the number of revisions. The socioeconomic burden is and will be immense [49–54].

This issue aims to address the cutting-edge topics concerning arthroplasty before, during and after surgery. It shows how surgeons are continuously looking for new ways to improve the outcomes for their patients and to share their knowledge with their community by sending these messages across as soon as possible so as to share innovation and improvements in care.

**Author Contributions:** All authors have read and agreed to the published version of the manuscript.

**Funding:** This research received no external funding.

**Conflicts of Interest:** The authors declare no conflict of interest.

## References

1. Beckmann, J.; Meier, M.K.; Benignus, C.; Hecker, A.; Thienpont, E. Contemporary knee arthroplasty: One fits all or time for diversity? *Arch. Orthop. Trauma. Surg.* **2021**, *141*, 2185–2194. [CrossRef] [PubMed]
2. Meier, M.; Janssen, D.; Koeck, F.X.; Thienpont, E.; Beckmann, J.; Best, R. Variations in medial and lateral slope and medial proximal tibial angle. *Knee Surgery, Sports Traumatol. Arthrosc.* **2020**, *29*, 939–946. [CrossRef] [PubMed]
3. Meier, M.; Zingde, S.; Best, R.; Schroeder, L.; Beckmann, J.; Steinert, A.F. High variability of proximal tibial asymmetry and slope: A CT data analysis of 15,807 osteoarthritic knees before TKA. *Knee Surgery Sports Traumatol. Arthrosc.* **2019**, *28*, 1105–1112. [CrossRef] [PubMed]
4. Meier, M.; Zingde, S.; Steinert, A.; Kurtz, W.; Koeck, F.; Beckmann, J. What Is the Possible Impact of High Variability of Distal Femoral Geometry on TKA? A CT Data Analysis of 24,042 Knees. *Clin. Orthop. Relat. Res.* **2019**, *477*, 561–570. [CrossRef] [PubMed]
5. Berichte | EPRD. Available online: https://www.eprd.de/de/downloads-1/berichte (accessed on 8 August 2022).
6. Beckmann, J.; Hirschmann, M.T.; Matziolis, G.; Holz, J.; Eisenhart-Rothe, R.V.; Becher, C. Recommendations for unicondylar knee replacement in the course of time: A current inven-tory. *Orthopade* **2020**, *50*, 104–111. [CrossRef]
7. Johal, S.; Nakano, N.; Baxter, M.; Hujazi, I.; Pandit, H.; Khanduja, V. Unicompartmental Knee Arthroplasty: The Past, Current Controversies, and Future Perspectives. *J. Knee Surg.* **2018**, *31*, 992–998. [CrossRef]
8. Klasan, A.; Tay, M.L.; Frampton, C.; Young, S.W. High usage of medial unicompartmental knee arthroplasty negatively influences total knee arthroplasty revision rate. *Knee Surg. Sports Traumatol. Arthrosc.* **2022**, *30*, 3199–3207. [CrossRef]
9. Hamilton, T.W.; Rizkalla, J.M.; Kontochristos, L.; Marks, B.E.; Mellon, S.; Dodd, C.A.; Pandit, H.G.; Murray, D.W. The Interaction of Caseload and Usage in Determining Outcomes of Unicompartmental Knee Arthroplasty: A Meta-Analysis. *J. Arthroplast.* **2017**, *32*, 3228–3237.e2. [CrossRef]
10. Thienpont, E.; Klasan, A. The dissatisfied total knee arthroplasty patient. New technologies-the white knight in shining armor coming to their rescue? *Arch. Orthop. Trauma. Surg.* **2021**, *141*, 2021–2025. [CrossRef]
11. Mathew, K.K.; Marchand, K.B.; Tarazi, J.M. Computer-Assisted Navigation in Total Knee Arthroplasty. *Surg. Technol. Int.* **2020**, *36*, 323–330.
12. Kayani, B.; Konan, S.; Ayuob, A.; Onochie, E.; Al-Jabri, T.; Haddad, F.S. Robotic technology in total knee arthroplasty: A systematic review. *EFORT Open Rev.* **2019**, *4*, 611–617. [CrossRef]
13. Liu, P.; Lu, F.-F.; Liu, G.-J.; Mu, X.-H.; Sun, Y.-Q.; Zhang, Q.-D.; Wang, W.-G.; Guo, W.-S. Robotic-assisted unicompartmental knee arthroplasty: A review. *Arthroplasty* **2021**, *3*, 15. [CrossRef] [PubMed]
14. Subramanian, P.; Wainwright, T.; Bahadori, S.; Middleton, R.G. A review of the evolution of robotic-assisted total hip arthroplasty. *HIP Int.* **2019**, *29*, 232–238. [CrossRef]
15. Jenny, J.-Y.; Picard, F. Learning navigation—Learning with navigation. A review. *SICOT-J* **2017**, *3*, 39. [CrossRef] [PubMed]

16. Siddiqi, A.; Horan, T.; Molloy, R.M.; Bloomfield, M.R.; Patel, P.D.; Piuzzi, N.S. A clinical review of robotic navigation in total knee arthroplasty: Historical systems to modern design. *EFORT Open Rev.* **2021**, *6*, 252–269. [CrossRef] [PubMed]
17. Rivière, C.; Iranpour, F.; Auvinet, E.; Howell, S.; Vendittoli, P.-A.; Cobb, J.; Parratte, S. Alignment options for total knee arthroplasty: A systematic review. *Orthop. Traumatol. Surg. Res.* **2017**, *103*, 1047–1056. [CrossRef]
18. Mariorenzi, M.; Levins, J.; Marcaccio, S.; Orfanos, A.; Cohen, E. Outpatient Total Joint Arthroplasty: A Review of the Current Stance and Future Direction. *Rhode Island Med. J.* **2013**, *103*, 63–67.
19. Pollock, M.; Somerville, L.; Firth, A.; Lanting, B. Outpatient Total Hip Arthroplasty, Total Knee Arthroplasty, and Unicompartmental Knee Arthroplasty: A Systematic Review of the Literature. *JBJS Rev.* **2016**, *4*, e4. [CrossRef]
20. Jaibaji, M.; Volpin, A.; Haddad, F.S.; Konan, S. Is Outpatient Arthroplasty Safe? A Systematic Review. *J. Arthroplast.* **2020**, *35*, 1941–1949. [CrossRef]
21. Vehmeijer, S.B.W.; Husted, H.; Kehlet, H. Outpatient total hip and knee arthroplasty. *Acta Orthop.* **2017**, *89*, 141–144. [CrossRef]
22. Husted, C.; Gromov, K.; Hansen, H.K.; Troelsen, A.; Kristensen, B.B.; Husted, H. Outpatient total hip or knee arthroplasty in ambulatory surgery center versus arthroplasty ward: A randomized controlled trial. *Acta Orthop.* **2019**, *91*, 42–47. [CrossRef] [PubMed]
23. Kremers, H.M.; Kremers, W.K.; Berry, D.J.; Lewallen, D.G. Social and Behavioral Factors in Total Knee and Hip Arthroplasty. *J. Arthroplast.* **2015**, *30*, 1852–1854. [CrossRef] [PubMed]
24. Hafkamp, F.J.; de Vries, J.; Gosens, T.; Oudsten, B.L.D. The Relationship Between Psychological Aspects and Trajectories of Symptoms in Total Knee Arthroplasty and Total Hip Arthroplasty. *J. Arthroplast.* **2020**, *36*, 78–87. [CrossRef]
25. Springer, B.D.; Sotile, W.M. The Psychology of Total Joint Arthroplasty. *J. Arthroplast.* **2020**, *35*, S46–S49. [CrossRef]
26. Siljander, M.P.; McQuivey, K.S.; Fahs, A.M.; Galasso, L.A.; Serdahely, K.J.; Karadsheh, M.S. Current Trends in Patient-Reported Outcome Measures in Total Joint Arthroplasty: A Study of 4 Major Orthopaedic Journals. *J. Arthroplast.* **2018**, *33*, 3416–3421. [CrossRef]
27. Haeberle, H.; Helm, J.M.; Navarro, S.; Karnuta, J.M.; Schaffer, J.L.; Callaghan, J.J.; Mont, M.A.; Kamath, A.F.; Krebs, V.E.; Ramkumar, P.N. Artificial Intelligence and Machine Learning in Lower Extremity Arthroplasty: A Review. *J. Arthroplast.* **2019**, *34*, 2201–2203. [CrossRef]
28. Gill, S.; Page, R. From big data to big impact: Realizing the potential of clinical registries. *ANZ J. Surg.* **2019**, *89*, 1356–1357. [CrossRef]
29. Bedard, N.A.; Pugely, A.J.; McHugh, M.A.; Lux, N.R.; Bozic, K.J.; Callaghan, J.J. Big Data and Total Hip Arthroplasty: How Do Large Databases Compare? *J. Arthroplast.* **2018**, *33*, 41–45. [CrossRef]
30. El-Galaly, A.; Grazal, C.; Kappel, A.; Nielsen, P.T.; Jensen, S.L.; Forsberg, J.A. Can Machine-learning Algorithms Predict Early Revision TKA in the Danish Knee Arthroplasty Registry? *Clin. Orthop. Relat. Res.* **2020**, *478*, 2088–2101. [CrossRef]
31. Wang, X.; Hunter, D.J.; Vesentini, G.; Pozzobon, D.; Ferreira, M.L. Technology-assisted rehabilitation following total knee or hip replacement for people with osteoarthritis: A systematic review and meta-analysis. *BMC Musculoskelet. Disord.* **2019**, *20*, 506. [CrossRef]
32. Varnum, C.; Pedersen, A.B.; Rolfson, O.; Rogmark, C.; Furnes, O.; Hallan, G.; Mäkelä, K.; de Steiger, R.; Porter, M.; Overgaard, S. Impact of hip arthroplasty registers on orthopaedic practice and perspectives for the future. *EFORT Open Rev.* **2019**, *4*, 368–376. [CrossRef] [PubMed]
33. Qasim, M.; Chae, D.S.; Lee, N.Y. Advancements and frontiers in nano-based 3D and 4D scaffolds for bone and cartilage tissue engineering. *Int. J. Nanomed.* **2019**, *14*, 4333–4351. [CrossRef] [PubMed]
34. Kwon, H.; Brown, W.E.; Lee, C.A.; Wang, D.; Paschos, N.; Hu, J.C.; Athanasiou, K.A. Surgical and tissue engineering strategies for articular cartilage and meniscus repair. *Nat. Rev. Rheumatol.* **2019**, *15*, 550–570. [CrossRef] [PubMed]
35. Weber, A.E.; Bolia, I.K.; Trasolini, N.A. Biological strategies for osteoarthritis: From early diagnosis to treatment. *Int. Orthop.* **2020**, *45*, 335–344. [CrossRef]
36. Kundu, S.; Ashinsky, B.G.; Bouhrara, M.; Dam, E.B.; Demehri, S.; Shifat-E-Rabbi, M.; Spencer, R.G.; Urish, K.L.; Rohde, G.K. Enabling early detection of osteoarthritis from presymptomatic cartilage texture maps via transport-based learning. *Proc. Natl. Acad. Sci. USA* **2020**, *117*, 24709–24719. [CrossRef]
37. Yu, C.; Zhao, B.; Li, Y.; Zang, H.; Li, L. Vibrational Spectroscopy in Assessment of Early Osteoarthritis—A Narrative Review. *Int. J. Mol. Sci.* **2021**, *22*, 5235. [CrossRef]
38. Onishi, O.; Ikoma, K.; Kido, M.; Kabuto, Y.; Ueshima, K.; Matsuda, K.-I.; Tanaka, M.; Kubo, T. Early detection of osteoarthritis in rabbits using MRI with a double-contrast agent. *BMC Musculoskelet. Disord.* **2018**, *19*, 81. [CrossRef]
39. Zarringam, D.; Saris, D.; Bekkers, J. The Value of SPECT/CT for Knee Osteoarthritis: A Systematic Review. *CARTILAGE* **2019**, *12*, 431–437. [CrossRef]
40. Wyngaert, T.V.D.; Palli, S.R.; Imhoff, R.J.; Hirschmann, M.T. Cost-Effectiveness of Bone SPECT/CT in Painful Total Knee Arthroplasty. *J. Nucl. Med.* **2018**, *59*, 1742–1750. [CrossRef]
41. Van der Bruggen, W.; Hirschmann, M.T.; Strobel, K.; Kampen, W.U.; Kuwert, T.; Gnanasegaran, G.; Van den Wyngaert, T.; Paycha, F. SPECT/CT in Postoperative Painful Hip Arthroplasty. *Semin. Nucl. Med.* **2018**, *48*, 439–453. [CrossRef]
42. Weber, M.-A.; Merle, C.; Rehnitz, C.; Gotterbarm, T. Modern Radiological Imaging of Osteoarthritis of The Hip Joint With Consideration of Predisposing Conditions. In *RöFo-Fortschritte auf dem Gebiet der Röntgenstrahlen und der bildgebenden Verfahren*; Georg Thieme Verlag KG: New York, NY, USA, 2016; Volume 188, pp. 635–651. [CrossRef]

43. Langer, R.; Vacanti, J. Advances in tissue engineering. *J. Pediatr. Surg.* **2015**, *51*, 8–12. [CrossRef] [PubMed]
44. Bakhshandeh, B.; Zarintaj, P.; Oftadeh, M.O.; Keramati, F.; Fouladiha, H.; Sohrabi-Jahromi, S.; Ziraksaz, Z. Tissue engineering; strategies, tissues, and biomaterials. *Biotechnol. Genet. Eng. Rev.* **2017**, *33*, 144–172. [CrossRef] [PubMed]
45. Koon, K.T.V.; Grenier, D.; Taborik, F.; Perrier, A.-L.; Mahieu-Williame, L.; Magnier, L.; Chuzel, T.; Contamin, H.; Chereul, E.; Beuf, O. Comparison of high-resolution magnetic resonance imaging and micro-computed tomography arthrography for in-vivo assessment of cartilage in non-human primate models. *Quant. Imaging Med. Surg.* **2021**, *11*, 3431–3447. [CrossRef] [PubMed]
46. Sun, Y.; Zuo, Z.; Kuang, Y. An Emerging Target in the Battle against Osteoarthritis: Macrophage Polarization. *Int. J. Mol. Sci.* **2020**, *21*, 8513. [CrossRef] [PubMed]
47. Jones, G.G.; Clarke, S.; Harris, S.; Jaere, M.; Aldalmani, T.; de Klee, P.; Cobb, J.P. A novel patient-specific instrument design can deliver robotic level accuracy in unicompartmental knee arthroplasty. *Knee* **2019**, *26*, 1421–1428. [CrossRef]
48. Fusco, G.; Gambaro, F.M.; Di Matteo, B.; Kon, E. Injections in the osteoarthritic knee: A review of current treatment options. *EFORT Open Rev.* **2021**, *6*, 501–509. [CrossRef]
49. Klug, A.; Gramlich, Y.; Rudert, M.; Drees, P.; Hoffmann, R.; Weißenberger, M.; Kutzner, K.P. The projected volume of primary and revision total knee arthroplasty will place an immense burden on future health care systems over the next 30 years. *Knee Surgery Sports Traumatol. Arthrosc.* **2020**, *29*, 3287–3298. [CrossRef]
50. Klug, A.; Pfluger, D.H.; Gramlich, Y.; Hoffmann, R.; Drees, P.; Kutzner, K.P. Future burden of primary and revision hip arthroplasty in Germany: A socio-economic challenge. *Arch. Orthop. Trauma. Surg.* **2021**, *141*, 2001–2010. [CrossRef]
51. Premkumar, A.; Kolin, D.A.; Farley, K.X.; Wilson, J.M.; McLawhorn, A.S.; Cross, M.B.; Sculco, P.K. Projected Economic Burden of Periprosthetic Joint Infection of the Hip and Knee in the United States. *J. Arthroplast.* **2020**, *36*, 1484–1489. [CrossRef]
52. Rak, D.; Weißenberger, M.; Horas, K.; von Hertzberg-Bölch, S.; Rudert, M. Mega-prostheses in revision knee arthroplasty. 2021, 50, 1011–1017. In *Der Orthopade*; Springer: Berlin/Heidelberg, Germany, 2021; Volume 50, pp. 1011–1017. [CrossRef]
53. Melnic, C.M.; Lightsey, H.M.; Calderón, S.A.L.; Heng, M. Megaprostheses in Nononcologic Hip and Knee Revision Arthroplasty. *J. Am. Acad. Orthop. Surg.* **2021**, *29*, e743–e759. [CrossRef]
54. Tarazi, J.M.; Chen, Z.; Scuderi, G.R.; Mont, M.A. The Epidemiology of Revision Total Knee Arthroplasty. *J. Knee Surg.* **2021**, *34*, 1396–1401. [CrossRef] [PubMed]

MDPI
St. Alban-Anlage 66
4052 Basel
Switzerland
www.mdpi.com

*Journal of Personalized Medicine* Editorial Office
E-mail: jpm@mdpi.com
www.mdpi.com/journal/jpm

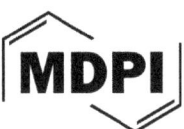

Disclaimer/Publisher's Note: The statements, opinions and data contained in all publications are solely those of the individual author(s) and contributor(s) and not of MDPI and/or the editor(s). MDPI and/or the editor(s) disclaim responsibility for any injury to people or property resulting from any ideas, methods, instructions or products referred to in the content.

www.ingramcontent.com/pod-product-compliance
Lightning Source LLC
LaVergne TN
LVHW070555100526
838202LV00012B/474